UNDER-EXPOSED

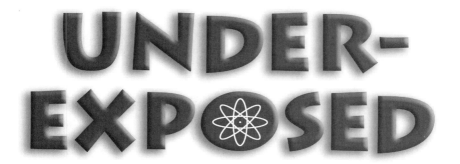

UNDER-EXPOSED

What If Radiation Is Actually

GOOD

for You ?

by Ed Hiserodt

Laissez Faire Books

a division of the Center for Libertarian Thought, Inc.

LITTLE ROCK, ARKANSAS

Laissez Faire Books is a division of
the Center for Libertarian Thought, Inc.
7123 Interstate 30, Suite 42
Little Rock, Arkansas 72209
www.LFB.com

ISBN 0-930073-35-5

Library of Congress Control Number: 2005931041

Printed in the United States of America

To Petr and Irene Beckmann
for their inspiration

and

to Kathleen Hiserodt
whose motivation and support
made this book a reality

Table of Contents

TABLES:

FIGURES:

Prologue

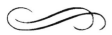

Radiation can be dangerous.
So can ignorance.

THE YOUNG WOMAN had injured her wrist in a fall, and the swelling would not go down. She made an appointment with her family physician to have an X-ray to determine if any bones had been broken. Several X-rays were taken to obtain different views. In a few minutes, they were developed, and the wrist was found to have a slight crack that required the use of a splint for several weeks.

In a few days, the young woman, already a mother, began to feel those subtle, suspicious changes in her body. She went again to the doctor to find she tested pregnant. But the memory of her X-ray haunted her. She knew that all radiation was harmful, and that it could cause her to have a retarded (or worse) baby. The next evening, she spoke with a nurse in her Women's Club who shared the same nuclear nightmare. The nurse suggested that she consider an abortion. A consultation with her gynecologist found him in agreement. The "therapeutic" abortion eliminated the possibility of a deformed baby.

This story was related to me by the woman, who by chance was reading the first draft of this book. I took her information to a health physicist I had met and asked him to estimate the amount of radiation the fetus would have received from the 1960s or 1970s X-ray machine—and what its likely effect would have been. In a few minutes he told me that the fetus would have received less than half the radiation received from a coast-to-coast airline flight, and that the effect would have been entirely negligible.

Radiation can be dangerous. So can ignorance.

I wonder what my niece or nephew would have been like. So does my sister.

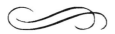

Chapter 1
Maybe What We Know Ain't So?

 *The trouble with people is not that they don't know,
but that they know so much that ain't so.*
—Josh Billings 1818–85

If you've been living on planet Earth anytime during the past fifty years, you are well aware of the dangers of radiation. We have learned that whenever we are exposed to X-rays, for example, there are certain precautions that must be taken. For dental X-rays, we'll need to have that lead-lined apron over us to make sure our reproductive organs are shielded from ionizing radiation. And, of course, the hygienist or technician must duck behind a lead partition because of the cumulative effect of any radiation that might bounce around the room. Not abiding by these rules will cause our cancer risk to increase substantially and may cause mutations in any children born after exposure of parental glands. All radiation is dangerous, and its danger is cumulative.

The thesis of this book contradicts such "common knowledge." While it is unquestionable that very high levels of radiation can cause death, illness, and the increased risk of cancer, there is unimpeachable evidence that *low levels* of radiation are not harmful to human life at all. In fact, we require *additional exposure* to ionizing radiation in order to achieve our optimum health and vitality.

It is my purpose in this book to convince you that:
- Low levels of ionizing radiation (that which we call "nuclear" or "atomic" radiation) are not harmful to human beings—or any other living creatures for that matter;
- With rare exceptions, we live in an environment where most of us could achieve *improved* health and vitality by increasing our exposure to radiation;

- While cancer is one of the three hazards of radiation (the other two being radiation sickness and death from huge doses), exposure to low levels of radiation would actually *reduce* occurrences of cancer; and
- Society is being denied a virtually unlimited source of clean energy with unimaginable benefits because of this irrational fear of radiation.

Certainly these statements may sound like the ravings of a mad man. I fully understand that and realize that it is up to me to provide adequate *evidence* to support my claims—which is mostly what this book is about. But first I'd like to lay a little groundwork, starting with a question that must be bothering you. "If low levels of radiation are not harmful and appear to be beneficial, why aren't scientists publishing papers about this and attempting to correct the public's misconceptions about radiation effects?"

That's an easy one. They are. And they too are amazed that what some see as "the story of the decade" is being totally ignored by the general media. Even those of us who diligently try to keep up with the news by reading a variety of news sources are unlikely to come across the subject (unless we are regular readers of *Health Physics* or *The Journal of Radiation Research*).

This book cites well over a hundred scientists—almost all with doctorates in their fields of specialty—that have published reams of data in more than fifty peer-reviewed scientific journals and scores of government documents. They are trying desperately to communicate their experimental results and the implications thereof to the public.

Many of them have not figured out that this is a *Green Issue* and that the reporters and editors are not about to go against their Green friends who reflexively demonize anything considered to be "pro-nuclear." But they're learning. If low levels of radiation are realized to be benign, then there goes the argument against nuclear power—and that may well tumble the house of cards that is the Green-Primitivists' argument against an industrialized society.

While there are, as mentioned, hundreds of scientists who are pushing for a truthful assessment of the effects of low levels of radiation, it was not always so. The one figure whose research in this area has been pivotal is Professor T.D. Luckey, now-retired chairman of the Biochemistry Department at the University of Missouri School of Medicine. His 1980 book *Hormesis with Ionizing Radiation*[1] cited more than a thousand experiments indicating that small amounts of radiation promoted growth and prolonged life in non-mammalian subjects. I can recall hearing of the book in 1981 and expecting a firestorm of interest in the beneficial uses of radiation. Not a word.

Dr. Luckey's second book, *Radiation Hormesis,*[2] is *the* seminal work on the subject of beneficial effects of radiation on humans and other mammals. By this time other researchers had concluded there was at least a threshold of radiation exposure below which there were no adverse effects. But Luckey would not back down from his hypothesis: that most of us require *additional* ionizing radiation for optimal health and well being. The evidence, as you will see, makes a compelling argument. But still not a word in the general media. It is from Luckey's second book that much of the material herein has been "harvested."

* * * * *

This book is about radiation hormesis—a phenomenon virtually unknown outside of certain scientific circles, but the understanding of which offers the potential for significant health benefits and a pathway to rational treatment of radiation dangers. By reopening access to the wonders of nuclear technology, it promotes a more abundant life for mankind. Since the radiation hormesis

[1] CRC Press, Boca Raton, Florida, 1980 (out of print).

[2] CRC Press, Boca Raton, Florida, 1991. Available from CRC Press, 2000 NW Corporate Blvd., Boca Raton, FL 33431, for $195 plus shipping.

hypothesis was put forth, it has caused a major upheaval in the scientific community about the effects of low-level radiation. At the same time, there has been an almost complete news blackout for the rest of us. I hope this book will help lift that veil.

The plan here is to provide you with information that helps cut through the confusing units of radiation intensity, its doses, the types of radiation, and other information that should allow you to make sense of the evidence. Then most of the book is in the form of evidence from experiments that were intended as studies of high-level effects, but in which the low-level data were also recorded. There are also several important investigations (with huge numbers of participants) where it was anticipated that the subjects would experience more cancer with an increase in radiation exposure, only to find that the exact opposite occurred.

At the outset you should know that there is nothing I can claim as original in the following pages. I am but an engineer reporting the results of scientists who have done the experiments or epidemiologists who have compiled and analyzed data related to the effects of low levels of exposure. Being free to "pick and choose," I've selected the studies I thought were most interesting and indicative of hormesis. However I did not exclude any because they showed opposite results. While I am certainly aware that there are many with *opinions* to the contrary, those who opine that low-level radiation is a danger have no data and must rely on extrapolations—and indeed, it is these very extrapolations that are the problem.

To Work, Dear Reader

You also have a job: It is to be totally skeptical of everything you read here. Doubt every sentence until I have presented sufficient evidence to back it up. There is an unbelievably large body of evidence about the effects of low doses of radiation on health, and some ninety-eight percent of it supports the hormesis model. I consider it quite an adventure to expose you to just a fraction of it.

Carefully and critically examine the evidence that is put forth here, and when you do, I believe that you will agree that the case I am making is indeed supported by the facts. And no longer will you allow the wool to be pulled over your eyes or those of your family, friends, and associates.

Let's begin by looking at how our attitudes toward radiation have changed during the past few decades.

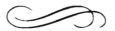

Chapter 2
I Still Have My Toes

We have got to stop science and scientific progress.... Facts separate people.
—Abby Hoffman

DATELINE: MEMPHIS, TENNESSEE; *circa 1950*: When my mother would take me to buy shoes in my pre-teen years, we would use the shoe store's fluoroscope to check the fit of shoes on my rapidly growing feet. I thoroughly enjoyed my chance to be like Superman with X-ray vision, seeing my toe bones wiggle through layers of rubber and canvas. Of course I would have to check several pairs of shoes each visit. And there were three or four visits every year.

DATELINE: EUROPE; *May 1986*: After the Chernobyl accident, there was, according to the International Atomic Energy Agency in Vienna, an increase of between 100,000 and 200,000 European babies who were intentionally aborted by their mothers. These were not unwanted fetuses. The babies' mothers had been convinced they might be carrying "nuclear monsters."

* * * * *

What is the significant of these two events, separated as they are in time and distance? In my opinion, they show the sea change in our attitude toward radiation dangers—and provide a good example of the widespread ignorance of the means and units by which dangers can be quantified.

While we'll get around to using proper units to describe radiation and its biological effects a little later, for now let's just call the radiation I got from inspecting my toes through the fluoroscope as *one SXR* (Shoe X-Ray.) We'll compare this dose to the doses received by the Europeans after Chernobyl.

Obviously the amount of radiation received from the accident at Chernobyl would be strongly dependent on geography. In Greece, where abortions were epidemic, the dose from Chernobyl was about 1.4 SXR units. This is the equivalent of the additional radiation received from background sources in nineteen months of living in Colorado instead of Texas. In Italy it was 0.8 SXR, in France less than 0.5 SXR. The increase over background radiation in Spain and Portugal was not really measurable, as the tiny theoretical increases disappeared below the slightest variations in natural background radiation.

So, what has changed in the forty-odd years since we didn't give a thought to using the shoe fluoroscope, and today, when mothers abort their children because of a mind-distorting fear that trivial amounts of radiation would cause genetic dangers to their *in utero* children? And we should remember, all of this occurred long after data were widely available showing no genetic damage or excessive mutations (over the approximately 6% rate of naturally occurring genetic defects) reported in extensive investigations of Japanese mothers exposed to *100,000 times* the radiation received by women downwind of the Chernobyl fire.

Before going on, though, let's look at the radiation on the borders of U.S. nuclear power plants, and also review the Three Mile Island "disaster" that anti-nuclear activists want so badly for us to consider as being on the same order of magnitude as Chernobyl.

Under U.S. law, it is the Nuclear Regulatory Commission (NRC) that regulates the amount of radiation that a nuclear power plant can emit annually at its boundary. In practice, the plants seldom approach this limit, but it amounts to just under 3% of a SXR. So, if you lived next to a power plant emitting its maximum for thirty-five years, you'd get the same amount of radiation I did each time I pushed the button to see if my Keds were large enough to be worn out before my toes pushed through.

"But what about accidents," you might ask, "such as the catastrophe at Three Mile Island?"

In our worst nuclear plant accident, the "survivors" living within a few miles of the "disaster" at TMI were subjected to a

The subject of radiation-causing mutations has been a favorite topic for cartoonist and comedy writers, as evidenced by the "Cone Heads" on *Saturday Night Live* and the brain-scrambled nuclear plant worker Homer Simpson. Only one problem: meticulous studies of the Japanese A-bomb survivors (over a fifty-plus-year period) have not uncovered any evidence of radiation-induced genetic abnormalities. But who cares about evidence?

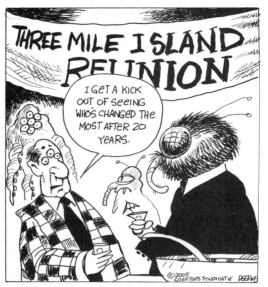

Cartoon reprinted with cartoonist John Deering's permission

withering 0.6% of an SXR—but only if they had remained un-clothed, outside, during the entire incident. Those who remained "on site" for the duration would have been exposed to just under one-half of an SXR.

But weren't there injuries at TMI? Only if you consider *anxiety* an injury. *All* the reported afflictions consisted of people who were either mentally or physiologically harmed by the media's sensationalistic mishandling of the incident. Ironically, those who evacuated to the homes of relatives in Denver would have received more additional radiation in a one-day stay than had they lain naked in the front yard of their Harrisburg homes during that week of media frenzy.[1]

---

[1] The main concern of the politicians and bureaucrats was a hydrogen bubble they feared would explode and spew radioactive materials across the area. Fortunately, there was a high-school chemistry student who reminded them that oxygen is needed for hydrogen combustion. The hydrogen was vented to the atmosphere, and the danger evaporated.

Falling for the Linear No-Threshold (LNT) Theory

Sadly, and ironically, the change in our attitudes toward radiation is due to an assumption—an assumption originally made to protect us from excessive exposure, but which has turned into the real "nuclear monster." We will examine it in detail later, but for now it might be best explained with an analogy to falling.

If we have found that falling 100 feet to a concrete floor is fatal in 100% of the cases and falling from fifty feet is fatal in 50% of them, we might logically expect the risk from falling twenty-five feet would result in a 25% death rate. But let's go on. At one foot, according to this "linear relationship between falling and death," we would expect one percent of the victims to die. At one inch, about 0.1%.

Yeah? Do you really think that out of 10,000 people who fall an inch, ten of them will die? If this linear relationship were the case, we would have thousands of people die every day from "falling" off their bathroom scales. Manhattan would have innumerable bodies in the street everyday from people "falling" off the curbs.

Everyone sees how ridiculous this "linear relationship" is in an activity like *falling* that we *know* about, yet we have been convinced to believe that this relationship is true for our response to ionizing radiation—a subject that very few of us understand. In later chapters we will look at the units that define radiation and how these compare to the "Linear No-Threshold" (LNT) theory of radiation at low doses—but first let's examine another scientific abomination.

Collective Dose

You are not going to believe a concept that has guided our radiation-protection formulators for the past forty or fifty years. But, as my hero Dave Barry would say, "I am not making this up." It's called *collective dose,* and it works like this: If 100 aspirins are a fatal dose for an individual, then when 100 people take one aspirin each, they have had a "collective dose" of 100 aspirins—therefore one of them is going to die. This is the reason you see all these dead people scattered all over the landscape… aspirin COD (Collective Over Dose).

It is *this exact concept* that has governed regulators in developing the "collective dose" policy that, in tandem with the LNT theory, has contributed to the regulatory madness of the EPA and NRC.

Since I suspect you still must think I'm putting you on about "collective dose," allow me to refer to page 10 in this very large, impressive volume on my desk—*The Health Physics and Radiological Health Handbook (Revised Edition).*[2] It shows the "Global Collective Dose" of carbon-14 released by the nuclear power industry to be 18,000 "person-Sieverts"—*a collective dose* measurement unit. What does that mean? It tells us that of the 6 billion people on earth exposed to these airborne emissions, 4.5 of them will die from the effects of carbon-14 emitted from nuclear power plants. How have we learned about these tragic deaths? Well, we *know* (from collective dose theory) that 4,000 person-Sieverts causes one excess death. So somewhere, some four and a half people on our terrestrial ball are going to die from this carbon-14 released from more than 440 power reactors.

Gee, could that be what did my grandmother in?

The average exposure here is less than 0.00003 SXR—an infinitesimally small amount, equivalent to a few minutes of normal background radiation. Yet, we are *told* that we should have faith in this unproven and unprovable theory—and to spend millions of our tax (or utility bill) dollars to save these 4.5 unfortunates who would otherwise be keeling over from this blast of searing radiation.

Time Out for a Measurement

Why, in a book about *hormesis* are we branching off into the areas of *Linear No-Threshold theory* and *collective dose*? Because the LNT and collective dose theories are both matters that directly affect public policy. Rules and laws are made on the basis of these

---

[2] Shielen, Bernard, ed., Scinta, Inc., Silver Spring, Md., 1992.

outmoded theories, and such restrictions stand in the way of any growth of marketplace interest in hormesis either as a therapy or as an immune-system stimulant. Advocates of hormesis—and you will see they are both numerous and impressive—consider burial of the LNT the first step toward public consideration and investigation of the hormesis phenomenon. Others, however, see this as the death knell of their domains. Let's see a few examples of the consequences from our present public policy.

Because They Say So, That's Why

The U.S. government plans to spend $85 billion (about $1,000 per U.S. family) in cleaning up a single radioactive site at Hanford, Washington—not to avoid the searing radiation analogous to falling 100 feet, but to escape the almost imperceptible disturbance from falling less than two-tenths of an inch. In terms of our SXR units, the Hanford reservation area (if you can find it in the Eastern Washington desert) has an annual "excessive" exposure of far less than 1 SXR, while it would take well over 6,000 SXR units to be fatal—and that would have to occur in a relatively short time or it might well be bio-positive. Alas long suffering taxpayers, I'm sorry to tell you that this is only one of four similar locations!

To these mega-clean-ups, you'll want to add the high cost of reducing the negligible emissions of nuclear plants, the counter-productive recommendations for reducing radon levels in homes, and last but not least—*Yucca Mountain,* the Federal government's potential (maybe someday in the future) high-level waste disposal site. In a move rivaling the building of Mayan pyramids to have a swell place to sacrifice virgins, Yucca Mountain is perhaps the greatest government boondoggle in U.S. history. Here we are spending billions of dollars to study outlandish fictions of (a) major climate changes bringing unprecedented rainfall to the desert where (b) the fictitious rain infiltrates through hundreds of feet of rock ordinarily considered impervious, to (c) dissolve stainless steel containers that hold the waste products after which they (d) seep through thousands of feet of rock into an isolated aquifer, into which (e) deep wells will be drilled that are impossible to drill without modern equipment, and (f) the water will be drunk by some unknown people who have modern drilling equipment, but no knowledge of any potential radiation danger. And that's the *reasonable* part of the Yucca Mountain story.

What is totally unreasonable is the contention that the so-called wastes would be harmful to anybody *after 10,000 years* no matter how they were eaten, drunk, sniffed, snorted, mainlined, or whatever. Nuclear medicine therapies routinely involve *millions* of times any conceivable exposure from this nuclear "seep-out." Government-paid, regulatory-agency-entrenched "scientists" are bewailing a potential tragedy caused by "high level" wastes that, in 600 to 1,000 years, will be less radioactive than the ores from which they came!

In addition to the wasting of taxpayer money—which we'll get back to in later chapters—the LNT theory has created irrational and unwarranted fears in citizens, causing them needless worry over their essential medical X-rays, tricking them into believing that irradiated foods are dangerous, and even causing unnecessary concern about 30,000 delayed cancer deaths predicted for their European relatives resulting from Chernobyl…which, incidentally, will most likely never happen, but wouldn't be detectable if they did.[3]

Lois, Call Clark!

All of this makes one continue to wonder: where are the journalists and the investigative reporters? They may not have taken biology and physics in college, but are they are unable to

---

[3] Evidence is (as you shall see) that there should be a decrease in the death rate in the higher ambient radiation areas. But, probably, we'll never be able to detect it. There would normally be approximately 25 million cancer deaths (plus or minus a few million) in the affected area. Thirty thousand additional would amount to a change of 0.1%—statistically undetectable. In the United States, cancer rates vary by about 50% between Utah (low) and the District of Columbia (high).

grasp the ramifications of changing the way radiation is viewed by major scientific organizations? Or do they think that their "environmentalist" buddies will get upset if they are involved in jerking a major plank out of the platform of those who want us to fear and distrust all technology? (What *would* the anti-nukes do if they couldn't scare Maude and Harry with stories of radioactive clouds and plutonium mega-deaths?)

Whatever the reason, a major discovery—that is inspiring a worldwide movement—has been totally ignored by the popular media. How important is the story? Myron Pollycove, M.D., Visiting Medical Fellow on the Nuclear Regulatory Commission, calls hormesis "the issue of the decade." As you will see, the evidence is incontrovertible. It is not challenged. It is ignored for whatever reason: ignorance, ideology, or indolence.

We have touched on what the taxpayers might save if the government policymakers were to understand that low-level radiation is harmless; but there are *positive* effects that those who have studied hormesis believe are even more compelling.

• **The potential benefits to health and vitality are phenomenal.** As we shall see, a random dosage of radiation reduced cancer mortality by forty percent in 15,000 nuclear workers, compared with their fellow workers who were not exposed. While cancer is the disease commonly associated with radiation—and consequently there are more data in this area of study—there was also a reduction of 26% in *deaths from all causes* in 28,542 exposed nuclear shipyard workers when weighed against co-workers with only normal background exposures. The latter investigation, which we will look at in some detail in chapter 19, indicates that there is a beneficial effect to the entire immune system, which, if properly understood and maximized, could lead to the reduction of infectious diseases and possibly prevention of immune-system dysfunctions.

• **Since the 1950s, uses of nuclear technology outside of medicine and industrial instrumentation have been stifled because of the fear of radiation.** (Smoke detectors are about the only consumer good that have escaped demonization by anti-nuclear activists because, in my opinion, they realized they could get annihilated by risk statistics on this one.)[4] What about community or even residential power plants taking advantage of the technology advances that have occurred over the past forty years? What about nuclear vehicles that would be fueled at the factory for twenty years?

The science for many nuclear miracles is either already available or within reach of technological development. But the pervasive fear of low levels of radiation keeps these advances from being used for the benefit of humanity.

• **For more than thirty years, the "energy crisis" has been a convenient excuse for those who want more government control over energy resources, but the "crisis" is phony as a three-dollar bill.** There is, and has been, readily available energy which is denied us solely because of the manufactured fear of low-level radiation.

This resource is not the *promise* of fusion, which seems to get further away every year, but the available-with-today's-technology breeder reactors that turn "wastes" into incredibly valuable fuel. Where, pray tell, do the advocates of environmentally pristine electric-powered vehicles think they are going to get the electricity to run those cute little things? A recent newspaper article warns that it would take at least a dozen full-scale (1,000-megawatt) power plants to replace the energy from gasoline and diesel engines in the transportation industry for the city of Los Angeles alone.

Available fuel from power plant "wastes" (which still have more than 95% of their original energy in a readily available form) and thousands of tons of "depleted" uranium currently choking our enrichment facilities could power the United States for many decades using available breeder reactor technology. Other uranium

---

[4] I recently found that Ralph Nader proved me wrong on this. He actually came out against smoke detectors because of the tiny speck of americium that has saved thousands of "real lives."

resources could fuel our country for centuries. But, as Edward Teller points out, the "breeding" of thorium—a source as common as dirt (actually it *is* dirt)[5]—into a useable fuel (Uranium 233) could easily provide energy for 100,000 years.

*   *   *   *   *

Radiation hormesis—just as in the case of nuclear power—will be opposed by radical "environmentalist" leaders who oppose *all* technological progress and the transfer of its benefits to the multitudes, whom they consider to be unwelcome intrusions on the "Green" concept of nature. But both hormesis therapy and nuclear energy will ultimately become commonplace in our world, because they are based on scientific truths that the doomsayers and propagandists can mask only for so long. The question is: "How much unnecessary human misery will occur before truth and reason prevail?"

So let's take a look at how we developed this fear of radiation.

---

[5] Each square mile of the earth's surface averages 2.5 tons of thorium in the first foot of depth.

Chapter 3
Radiation: Fears Versus Reality

 *Some observers believe there will be a million people with direct and backup assignments to guard the nuclear industry by the year 2000.*
—Ralph Nader, 1975

M OST PEOPLE BELIEVE that radiation—the kind that comes from nuclear power plants—is not only dangerous, but cumulatively so. A little now, a bit more later—it all adds up with life-threatening consequences. We have been convinced over many years that all radiation has the ability to cause cancer, and the more we get of it, the more likely we are to develop the disease. There is also a prevalent idea that radiation causes mutations in humans because of its damage to our DNA. (This will also be shown to be false, even when the radiation levels are very high, as in the Japanese cities bombed at the end of World War II.)

So how did we come to "know" these things? Where did we get our fear of radiation? That's an interesting question.

It's not one of those innate fears like the fear of heights or growling animals. How could we be born with a fear of something we can't feel, smell, see, or otherwise sense?

It's not something your parents taught you. Did your mother ever say, "Darling, be sure to look both ways when you cross the street, and watch out for gamma rays"?

I suggest that our fear of radiation comes from two sources. First is its invisibility and lack of any kind of "early warning" alerting us to a dangerous presence. If gamma radiation were seen as purple flashing lights, we could see its presence and avoid it, much as many of us must do to prevent being sunburned. In this way radiation is similar to the plague and other scary germ-borne diseases: We tend to fear any kind of invisible killer—as well we should. Being rational beings, however, we don't stay inside under oxygen tents because the Ebola virus is active in Africa or because a Nile virus-bearing mosquito *might* be in the neighborhood. We make a "risk versus benefit" analysis in order to live a normal life, and we save our irrationality for radiation.

The second reason is an almost total lack of knowledge of radiation, how it is measured, and its effects at various levels. The common knowledge is that all radiation is dangerous, period. Most science textbooks don't add much, if anything, to this dearth of knowledge. Typically there will be a picture of a nuclear plant with a caption reading: "Concrete and steel walls four to five feet thick protect workers from deadly radiation." If we were to see a newspaper article stating that "Mrs. Jones is wearing a special protective suit to ward off the poison darts," we would rush to the next paragraph to find out what kind of darts? How many? How poisonous? Where are they coming from? But as regards nuclear "darts," we just nod our heads and think, "Well, all radiation is dangerous."

A "Media Created" Fear?

Dr. Bernard Cohen—who was group leader for cyclotron research at Oak Ridge about the same time I was researching my toes in the shoe store X-ray machine—had noticed a disparity between the deaths and injuries from radioactivity accidents and the media's concern over this danger. So, like the researcher he is, he obtained the number of entries in the *New York Times* Information Bank for the years 1974–1978 for various types of accidents and the death toll resulting from them.[1] (This avoided the Three Mile Island "disaster," which would have made the situation look much more ridiculous than it already does.) His data looked like Table 1.

This table reminded me of two news stories I read less than a month apart some years ago, both of which reported more than twenty deaths in two separate geothermal well accidents in South

---

[1] Bernard Cohen, *The Nuclear Energy Option,* Plenum Press, New York, 1990, pp. 58–59.

Table 1 News Stories on Deaths from Various Causes

	News Stories	Deaths Per Year	In Previous Decade
Auto accidents	120	50,000	500,000
Industrial accidents	50	12,000	120,000
Asphyxiation accidents	20	4,500	45,000
Radiation accidents	200	0	0

Source: New York Times Information Bank, 1974–1978.

America. Do you remember them? Or the dozens killed in refinery accidents and pipe line accidents? How about the 100 people that are killed each year from being hit by trains carrying coal for power generation? I guess those people are not as important as the people who didn't lose their lives in nuclear accidents.

Just How Dangerous Is Radiation?

In March 1954, sailors onboard the *Lucky Dragon* were exposed to fallout from a hydrogen bomb test conducted on Bikini atoll. While his two compatriots suffered from radiation sickness, one sailor died the following September. I was a teenager at this time, and yet I can remember a huge amount of news regarding the incident. I suspect it shaped my fear of radiation.

In July 2000, a joint U.S.-Russian Federation report gave as sixty the total number of "criticality" accidents that had occurred in the United States, Russia, France, the United Kingdom, Canada, Argentina, and Japan. These accidents occur when too much "fissionable" material comes together for whatever reason and produces for a few moments the same conditions as would be found inside a nuclear reactor. It doesn't cause a "nuclear explosion" but a flash of blue light and a large spike of heat energy. Mr. Harry Daghlian has the unenviable distinction of being the first criticality accident victim in August 1945, during the Manhattan project. Since then, there have been twenty-one similar deaths, with seven having occurred in the United States.

The most recent were in 1999 when an accident at a Japanese enrichment facility killed two workers. A third worker survived after experiencing severe radiation sickness. I saved the newpaper with that story (prior to the deaths) with the headline "Japanese contain radioactive gas leak" emblazoned across five of six columns at the top of the front page. On the same page there was a notice "Deadly quake strikes Mexico/Page 7A." Oh well, I guess earthquake deaths just aren't fashionable.

Yes, sadly some individuals have died from exposure to radiation. But it is surprising how few, and since there are so few we can account for all or nearly all of them. (This obviously doesn't count the unfortunates who were victims at Hiroshima and Nagasaki, almost all of whom died from blast and heat, but would very likely have died of radiation sickness had they survived the primary causes.)

It is unclear what killed the thirty-one firemen and rescue workers at the Chernobyl disaster. The graphite reactor was in flames (not possible in U.S. power reactors) and was convecting extremely radioactive materials from the core. The probable cause of the firemen's death was heat, since death by radiation generally takes several days to do its work on internal organs. But they, as in the case of the Japanese bomb victims, would very likely have died from radiation.[2]

Unclean!

On September 13, 1987, two thieves entered an abandoned clinic in Goiania, State of Goia, Brazil, and dismantled a machine used for radiation therapy. From it they took a stainless steel cylinder, which they broke apart with a sledge hammer and then

---

[2] I cannot allow Chernobyl to be considered in the same light as other nuclear power facilities. It was built by a Communist government with no concern for the safety of its citizens—as evidenced by the lack of a containment structure to prevent what did happen from happening—and constructed with graphite, rather than water, as a moderator in order that it could be used to produce bomb-grade plutonium. In my opinion, the firemen were murdered by a lack of responsibility on the part of the Soviet government.

sawed open a one-cubic-inch capsule filled with a glittering powder—cesium 137...1250 curies of it. Children in the junkyard began to play with it, and the workers took some home with them. Two weeks later, four people died, one was to have his arm amputated, and several skin grafting operations were required for those having had intimate contact with the highly radioactive isotope.

Four deaths from fire, traffic, or a trench collapsing might have been totally overlooked by the news. But death by radiation is our modern-day leprosy. Fear of radioactive contamination caused the wholesale value of the entire agricultural production of the state to fall by 50%. Vacationers, afraid of the "invisible killer," cancelled 40% of the hotel rooms booked for the tourist season; conventions were moved to other states or called off. Hotels in other parts of the country refused to register Goians, while airline pilots and taxi drivers denied them transportation. Cars with Goiania license plates were stoned.

Of the 125,000 individuals who insisted on a Geiger scan, 8.3% showed signs of acute stress (extreme anxiety, rashes, vomiting, diarrhea) from fear—yet not one was found contaminated. The funeral of the first victim had to be delayed while police stopped the stoning and removed barricades at the cemetery. Where did this paralyzing fear of radiation come from? I would suspect that the Goian newspapers printed stories similar to those noted in Bernard Cohen's table of *New York Times* stories, resulting in similar attitudes toward the dangers of radiation.

The Radiation Death Toll

The total number of people known (or suspected by me) to have been killed directly by exposure to radiation is:
- One fisherman killed by bomb-test fallout
- Twenty-two killed in criticality accidents
- Four killed in Goia, Brazil
- Thirty-one murdered by the Soviets (yes, I do have a grudge)

A total of fifty-eight have died, or may have died, from direct exposure to radiation in about the same number of years with a world average population of around 4 billion. Five of these were members of the "general public." I may have missed a few, but the point is that, statistically, death from direct exposure to radiation is about as likely as death from the bite of a rabid cow.

What if we were to confront an anti-nuclear activist from the grossly misnamed "Union of Concerned Scientists" or the Sierra Club with this statistic? Would they deny it? Oh, maybe they would say that a fisherman on another boat at another time was a fallout victim, but in general this would not be of any concern to them. What would be important to them is the number of deaths that occurred "that we don't know about but are scientifically calculated."

A Slippery Slope

When we read the statistics on deaths involving automobile accidents, we are given the actual count of deaths as compiled by various law enforcement agencies. But when the anti-nuclear zealots tell us about the number of people who died as a result of radiation from exposure to, say, radon, they don't have a single victim they can point to with any degree of certainty. Their "statistical deaths" come from an extrapolation based on the Linear No-Threshold (LNT) theory. Just as with our falling analogy, they correctly note that very high exposures, like falling from very tall buildings, increase the likelihood of death (by cancer, in the case of radiation). Their argument falls apart when they try to extend, or extrapolate, the high-dose exposure to much lower exposures.

For a moment, let's jump to an example detailed in a later chapter. Studies of the Japanese indicated that exposure to the equivalent of 100 SXR units (20 rem, if you're ahead of me) in a short time would double the number of leukemia deaths in a population of one million people, from the expected fifty deaths to one-hundred. The LNT extrapolation would predict one-tenth the increase in deaths (in this case, five) if the population were exposed to one-tenth that additional exposure (in this case, 10 SXR units).

Could they point to any bodies? No, they only have their theoretical corpses *based on the LNT extrapolation.* But in this case, there is *actual data that completely contradict the LNT theory's prediction.* Not only did the death rate *not* increase; it actually *decreased*— by an astounding 40%! To summarize:

- **Fifty** deaths expected in unexposed population
- **Fifty-five** deaths predicted by LNT extrapolation
- Only **thirty** deaths occurred, according to actual data

*   *   *   *   *

Therein lies the crux of the hormesis/LNT controversy: Those who advocate the Linear No-Threshold theory base their *belief* on the extrapolation of high-level exposure responses down to low levels. But when low-level data are available, they almost always show a bio-positive—or stimulatory—response. It is this response, called *hormesis,* that we will be discussing in the next chapter.

Chapter 4
Hormesis—Grasping the Concept

The dose makes the poison.
—Tenet of Pharmacology

Hormesis derives from the Greek *hormo* meaning "I excite" from which we also get the word *hormone*. While of classic origin, *hormesis* has only recently found its way into many dictionaries and seems to have had its first modern usage by C.M. Southam and J. Erlich in a 1943 study of fungi reported in an unpronounceable scientific journal.[1] The word refers to a phenomenon stated by the "Arndt-Schulz" Law:

Small doses of poison are stimulatory.

Rudolf Arndt (a psychiatrist) and Hugo Schulz (a pharmacologist) were nineteenth-century German researchers who diluted poisons to the point that they were not only no longer poisonous, but had a positive effect on the growth and reproductive rates of yeast. For example, when mercury chloride is diluted by a factor of 700,000, it becomes a stimulant for bacterial growth instead of an extremely potent germicide. Arsenious acid, poisonous to bacteria in normal concentrations, showed a positive effect when diluted by 40,000 times its volume. The Arndt-Schulz team demonstrated that their principle was—or at least appears to be—universal, with regard to the dilution of inorganic toxins.

While Arndt-Schulz seem to be the first to *quantify* the "low-dose" effect of chemical poisons, the phenomenon had been described earlier by Bernard in *Repair Strengthens Tissue* (1867), by

---

[1] OK, you try it: *Phytopathology*. The full citation is "Effects of extract of western red-cedar heartwood on certain wood decaying fungi in culture." Vol. 33, p. 517, 1943.

Hahnemann in *Homeopathic Medicine* (1810), and even earlier by a Swiss physician and chemist, Philippus Aureolus Paracelsus,[2] in *The Dose Is Everything* (1520).

A relatively modern work on the subject, *The General Adaptive Syndrome,* was written by Nobel Laureate Hans Seyle in 1944. While he identified many agents that increased the resistance of the host to disease, his primary emphasis was on the effects of stress— both the excessive mind-destroying stress of battle and his observation that little is accomplished by humans unless there is some minimal amount of stress-stimulation in their lives. Seyle's contention was that minute doses of the hormetin (the hormetic or stimulatory agent) start an *alarm reaction,* small doses induce the *stage of resistance,* and still larger doses bring about a *stage of exhaustion* in which the organism is no longer able to cope with the stressing agent. X-rays were one of the stress agents he often mentioned.[3]

Walter A. Heiby shows numerous examples of low-dose stimulation—and the problem of over-stimulation—in his 1988 book, *The Reverse Effect: How Vitamins and Minerals Promote Health and CAUSE Disease.*[4] As you may have already deduced, his term for hormesis is "the reverse effect," expressing the change in response due to different levels of the same stimulant.

Prior to Southam and Erlich's use of the word *hormesis* in 1943 and Luckey's subsequent popularization of the term in his 1980 and 1991 books, another even worse tongue-torturer was used to characterize the phenomena: *hormoligosis*—which better defines the action of a small dose from the Greek *olig* meaning small or few, as in *oligarchy.*

---

[2] His real name was Theophrastus Bombastus von Hohenheim. (Somehow I think I could have come up with an easier *nom de plume.*) Aside from his work in chemistry, he is credited with being the first to point out the relation between goiter in the parent and cretinism in the child.

[3] In describing his experiments, Sele remarked, "I could find no noxious agent that did not elicit the syndrome"—meaning, of course, the "reverse effect."

4 MediScience Publishers, Dearfield, Ill., 1988. Available for $59.50 from MediScience Publishers, Box 256A, Dearfield, IL 60015.

Hormetins

While we will be concerned with hormesis arising from exposure to ionizing radiation, this is only one area where the phenomenon is exhibited.[5] Other *physical* "hormetins" include gravity, pressure, sound, heat, motion, time, magnetism, light, and certain other frequencies of electromagnetic radiation. Each of these—in low amounts—can stimulate the vitality of living organisms but causes harm or death to the organism in much higher dosages. That ionizing radiation does likewise is not the peculiarity; it would be much more unusual if it didn't.

Among the more important *chemical* hormetic agents are the metal ions (e.g., germanium, mercury, lead, tin, and cadmium), oxygen, fluorine, arsenic, and selenium. While our protectors at the Environmental Protection Agency (EPA) would croak if they could detect some of these elements in *any* quantity whatsoever, they (the trace elements, not the EPA) are necessary for our optimum heath and vitality.

Organic chemical hormetins include antibiotics, insecticides, vitamins, certain nutrients, some food additives, many drugs, and free radicals. It should be noted that many hormetic effects are anything but subtle. When crickets were fed $1/100$ the fatal dose of the insecticide *chlordane,* they grew to be twice (!) as large as their unpoisoned cohorts.[6] (I think our mosquitoes may be eating this stuff.)

I must tread lightly when it comes to claims of *biologic* initiators of hormesis—since I have only the vaguest idea of what they are, and virtually no idea of how they act to stimulate the organism.

---

[5] Luckey's first book, *Hormesis with Ionizing Radiation,* was initially a survey of various hormetic agents and their effects. When he came to ionizing radiation, there was so much material that his wife convinced him to write the book specifically on that topic. (As is usual in marriages, *she* had the idea, but *he* took the credit!)

[6] *Insecticide Hormoligosis,* J. Economic Entomology, February 1968. This article, along with *Hormoligosis in Pharmacology,* J. Am. Medical Assoc., 173: 1960, appear to be part of Luckey's preparation for recognizing effects of radiation hormesis.

They, however, are known (by other people) to include hormones (naturally), cytokines, enzyme cofactors, cell maturation compounds, and nerve transmission compounds. These are also known as *intra-organismic* agents. But wait, there's more …

There are also *inter-organismic* hormetins, such as pheromones, which are even more confusing—at least to me. And these lead us to the most puzzling agents of all: socio-psychologic factors … including stress, love, sex, hate, responses to crowding, and fear. One can begin to see why Dr. Luckey's wife advised him to stick to something simple, like hormesis from ionizing radiation.

Hormesis—A Little Deeper

The primary tenet of hormesis is contained in a cardinal rule of pharmacology: The poison is in the dose.[7]

Figure 1 gives a graphical representation of this postulate. Point A on the curve represents a "normal" amount of something—

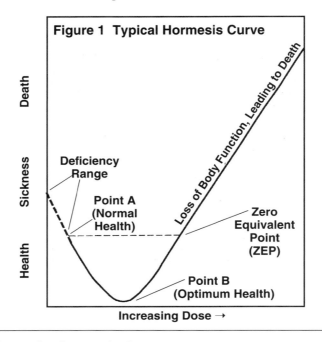

Figure 1 Typical Hormesis Curve

---

[7] Often stated as *The Dose Makes the Poison.*

let's use, for example, Vitamin A—which results in what we might call "normal healthfulness." Less than this dose (the dashed line) will move us up into the "unhealthy" zone, making us prone to deficiency diseases such as night blindness. As we take more of the supplement, there is—assuming the vitamin companies aren't lying to us—an increase in the health benefit … until we reach point B.

At this *inflection point,* a dramatic change occurs: Up to this point, the more of the vitamin, the healthier; but from here on, the more we take, the *less healthy,* since we have passed the optimum dose. If we continue to take more, we reach a point at which the dose provides us the same level of health we would have had if we had not taken *any* additional Vitamin A: the Zero Equivalent Point (ZEP). From here on out, though, the news gets worse: More makes us sick; still more kills us.

Hold on now. If we shift our definitions just a little bit, we can call poisons such as selenium "necessities"—since they are necessary for optimum health—and necessities such as salt "poisons." It is merely a matter of degree, is it not? Salt fits the same curve as Vitamin A and arsenic. Too little salt, unhealthiness (or possible death); too much salt, unhealthiness (and certain death.) It's as if: *The dose makes the poison!* Or maybe:

All things are poison; nothing is poison.

This illustrates one of the problems with explaining—and understanding—hormesis: It is counterintuitive. We naturally tend to think in terms of less-poison-good, more-poison-bad. Just-a-tiny-bit-of-poison-good, doesn't figure in.

Adding a bit to our confusion is the shape of the hormesis curve. Our "vitamin example" is oriented with "unhealthiness" in the upward, or positive, direction. This is done for compatibility with the convention for carcinogen-response curves. As we shall see, many other plots have the beneficial effect in the "up" direction.

While we're looking at the hormesis curve, we might as well take a look at the other theories of dose-response in comparison, as shown in Figure 2. The LNT is linear, as we would expect from its name, and indicates that all exposure is cumulatively dangerous. We often see this dose-response relationship for high levels of toxins such as lead.[8] The *threshold* plot shows no effect from the agent at low doses; but at some threshold value of dose, the health effect becomes negative. We see this response to such substances as caffeine. (Even here we would likely get arguments that in small doses caffeine has beneficial properties.) When one starts searching for examples of threshold effects, the much more prevalent hormetic examples keep getting in the way.

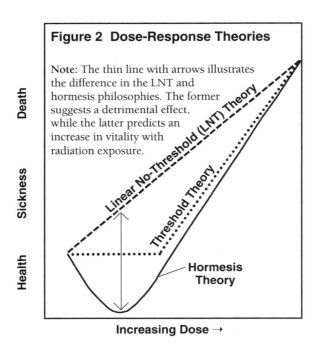

Figure 2 Dose-Response Theories

Note: The thin line with arrows illustrates the difference in the LNT and hormesis philosophies. The former suggests a detrimental effect, while the latter predicts an increase in vitality with radiation exposure.

Linear No-Threshold (LNT) Theory

Threshold Theory

Death

Sickness

Health

Hormesis Theory

Increasing Dose →

---

[8] It wouldn't surprise me if lead had some sort of a threshold also, but it is generally considered to have a cumulatively harmful effect.

Before Going on to Radiation…

Let's look at some common examples of where we see hormesis in humans.

- Vitamins and trace minerals clearly show the difference a dose makes. Arsenic and selenium were considered (and are) deadly poisons; but they have been found to be necessary nutrients.
- Some sunlight is necessary for production of vitamin D in the body, but too much leads to localized cancers, and, in extreme cases, death.
- Some noises (such as waves) can be soothing and healthful, while long exposure to loud noises can cause mental confusion and loss of hearing function.
- Most athletes are well aware of "no pain, no gain;" too much pain, however, equals ruptured muscles, torn ligaments, and broken bones.
- Lack of stress in one's life (e.g., a deadline to complete a project) tends to make an individual lethargic, while too much stress can cause permanent physical and mental harm.

We'll be going on shortly to the specifics of *radiation hormesis,* but first, classes on the basics of ionizing radiation are getting under way in the next chapter.

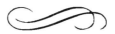

Chapter 5
Introduction to Remedial Nuclear Physics

Atom: from the Greek atomos
meaning indivisible

Most of us are familiar with the representation of the atom shown in Figure 3, proposed by Niels Bohr in 1913: a nucleus orbited by electrons. While there have been many major additions to our knowledge about the atom over the past hundred years, the Bohr model still provides a convenient way to look at the atom—

Figure 3 Representation of Carbon 12 Atom

The carbon atom has 6 protons and 6 electrons giving it an **atomic number** of 6. *Most* carbon atoms have 6 neutrons which, when added to the protons, give it an average **atomic weight** of about 12.

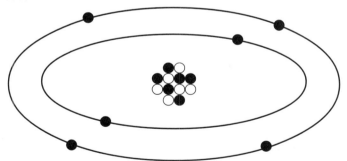

If the atom were drawn to scale with the orbits (or fields) of the electrons being the size of an average bedroom, the electrons would be microscopic, while the nucleus would be about the size of a pin head. It is only in the tiny nucleus that atomic phenomena (such as radioactivity) occur.

On the other hand, chemical properties of an element are related to its atomic number (the number of protons)—although it is actually the electrically counteracting electrons that share orbits (or fields) with other elements to make chemical compounds.

---

even though it was originally missing one major component (the neutron), which we'll get to in a moment.

During the early twentieth century, a number of physical chemists worked on the relationships between the elements. Hydrogen was, by then, known to be the lightest of the elements and uranium thought to be the heaviest. In 1907, J.J. Thompson constructed an apparatus to measure the relative weights of the elements—and ran into a problem. The weights of the elements did not correspond to the integers used to classify their position on the table of elements. Moreover, he found some atoms that seemed to have two (or more) different weights according to his "mass spectrometer." Neon, for instance, was found to have two weights—20 and 22—when compared with the weight of a hydrogen atom.

In 1932, spurred on by his mentor, Ernest Rutherford, James Chadwick of Cambridge University discovered the existence of the neutron, an atomic particle with the same weight as the proton, but without an electrical charge. It soon became clear that, while elements were identified (and reacted chemically) by their number of protons, many had differing numbers of neutrons. These variations became known as **isotopes**.[1]

It is important to note that the **atomic number** of an element is equal to the number of protons in the nucleus, while the **atomic weight** is the sum of the protons *and* neutrons.

Because isotopes have different numbers of neutrons, most atomic weight figures in the periodic table are not integers, but a weighted average of the atomic weights of all the isotopes of that element. We'll be using two conventions to denote the atomic weight of an isotope. For example, a carbon atom with eight neutrons (and its mandatory six protons, if it is to be carbon) will be written simply as carbon 14 or, alternatively, with the atomic weight superscript writ-

---

[1] Actually the word *isotope* had been coined by Nobel laureate Frederick Soddy almost twenty years earlier; he just didn't know why they existed until the discovery of the neutron.

ten before the elemental symbol, as in "^{14}C." (You may find in other literature that the superscript appears after the element symbol.)

Hydrogen offers a simple example of isotopes. Figure 4 shows three forms of the element: The first is just regular[2] hydrogen, designated as H or ^1H, which has one proton and no neutrons. The second form, *deuterium* or ^2H, is known as "heavy hydrogen."[3] It

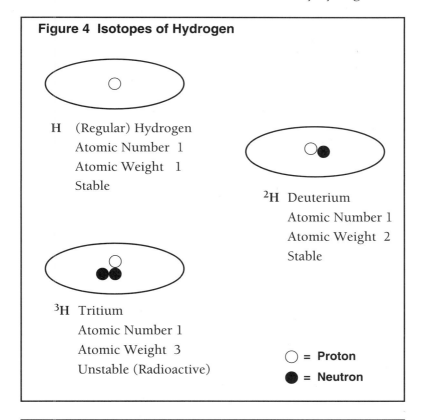

Figure 4 Isotopes of Hydrogen

H   (Regular) Hydrogen
    Atomic Number 1
    Atomic Weight 1
    Stable

^2H Deuterium
    Atomic Number 1
    Atomic Weight 2
    Stable

^3H Tritium
    Atomic Number 1
    Atomic Weight 3
    Unstable (Radioactive)

○ = **Proton**
● = **Neutron**

---

[2] It has a name, *protium*, but it's only used by real physics nerds or trivia freaks.

[3] Deuterium is the form of hydrogen that makes "heavy water," the substance on which many World War II spy novels are based. These stories are based on a factual February 1943 raid on the heavy water concentration plant operated by the Nazis in Vemork, Norway. While an earlier attempt resulted in disaster—all thirty-four commandos were either killed in glider crashes or executed by the Germans—the second raid was a textbook example of guerrilla warfare and bravery. Disabling the Vemork plant was a major setback for the Axis A-bomb program.

has the obligatory single hydrogen proton, but also has a neutron in its nucleus. Finally, the form of hydrogen known as *tritium,* or ^{3}H, is seen to have two neutrons.

All three forms are known as *isotopes* with ^{1}H making up 99.98% of the total hydrogen that we know about—and presumably in the universe. Both "regular" hydrogen and deuterium are **stable** isotopes, meaning that they don't change over time.

But tritium is another story: it is an **unstable** isotope[4] that will eventually **decay** or **disintegrate** into stable ^{1}H. It is this process—where atoms go to pieces—that we normally call **radioactivity**.

About three-fourths of the elements have two or more stable isotopes and many have radioactive (unstable) ones, some of which can be useful, and others of which can be dangerous if we come into contact with them. A few of the more common radioactive isotopes and beneficial uses are noted in Table 2.

Table 2 Some Common Radioactive Isotopes

^{3}H	Tritium	Luminous watch dials
^{14}C	Carbon 14	Radioactive dating
^{60}Co	Cobalt 60	Food irradiation
^{40}K	Potassium 40	Biological tracer
^{99}Tc	Technetium 99	Medical diagnosis
^{131}I	Iodine 131	Thyroid-function diagnosis and treatment
^{238}Pu	Plutonium 238	Spacecraft power supplies, pacemakers
^{241}Am	Americium 241	Smoke alarms

---

[4] All tritium eventually undergoes "beta-decay" in which the neutron changes into a proton and an electron—a feat of amazing atomic legerdemain.

All of the elements heavier than lead in the periodic table have multiple isotopes, and all are naturally radioactive; most of them decay into one of the stable lead isotopes. Uranium and thorium have the greatest number of isotopes—uranium with 22 isotopes and thorium with 28—though most of these are not naturally occurring. As a rule of thumb, elements are happiest when they have about the same number of protons and neutrons. When there is a sizable difference, they tend to decay until there isn't.

So, what about this radioactive business? How does it work? How dangerous is it? And for how long?

A very interesting subject: Don't miss the next chapter.

Chapter 6
Types of Ionizing Radiation

 *There is no amount of radiation that is safe.*
—Anti-nuclear activist Dr. John Gofman

WHEN A RADIOACTIVE isotope decays, it emits one or more of three forms of ionizing radiation: alpha particles, beta particles, or gamma rays. One problem in discussing the effects of radiation is the lack of understanding of these different types and how they affect the body.

Alpha-particles are actually helium nuclei, which can be seen from the periodic table to have an atomic number of two and an atomic weight of four.[1] In the subatomic world, the emission of an alpha-particle is like shooting a shot put with a sling shot: there is a lot of mass involved, but it doesn't travel very far. This particle gives up its considerable energy in one-half to two inches of air. It can't penetrate the skin and, consequently, isn't dangerous when outside the body. Because of its mass, however, it is considered to be quite dangerous[2] when inside the body—particularly when inhaled, where it may remain in the lungs in close proximity to lung tissue cells for extended periods. Fortunately, there are some very good data on this subject that we'll look into.

Beta-particles are high energy electrons that can penetrate up to three feet of air, or the first layer of skin cells, and can cause a burn not unlike that from falling asleep in the tanning bed. Beta-burns were a particular problem for workers after the Chernobyl chemical explosion and for technicians involved in some phases of

---

[1] In alpha-decay, the radioactive isotope is changed to the isotope of an element with an atomic number two less and an atomic weight four less than the original element.

[2] It is *common knowledge* that plutonium, an alpha emitter, is deadly when inhaled. You will see in chapter 16 that *common knowledge* may be terribly mistaken.

the weapons-testing program in Nevada. With a mass some $1/7344$ that of an alpha particle, its energy is derived from its speed, which can approach 99.8% of the speed of light. Relatively speaking, beta "rays" are not considered much of a threat to human health although there can be complications arising from beta-burns.

A third possible product from the decay of a radionuclide (a fancy word for a radioactive isotope) is **gamma radiation**, which is considered to be the greatest danger from nuclear decay. It is very similar—in fact in some cases identical—to X-rays and can penetrate several feet of concrete or inches of steel. Like any other electromagnetic radiation, its intensity falls off as the square of the distance from the source. For instance, the exposure at 100 yards is $1/900$ that at 10 feet; at a quarter mile, the radiation is reduced by a factor of 17,424 compared with the 10-foot value.[3]

There are other forms of radiation that should be mentioned even though they are not the normal products of natural decay. The first is **cosmic radiation**. It consists of various types of particles, sub-particles, and high-energy photons arriving on Earth from every direction in the cosmos. Cosmic radiation, with both solar and galactic components, can have unbelievably high energies, but, fortunately, it poses no danger, since there is so little of it. For instance, protons that originated in far-off galaxies four billion years ago have energies 100 million times greater than can be created in our most advanced particle accelerators. But only about one of these per year is detected by the Akeno Giant Air Shower Array located just west of Tokyo.[4]

These cosmic sources make up less than 10% of the background radiation that the average U.S. citizen receives, yet we still

---

[3] Luckey mentions another form of radiation, *delta rays,* with low energies and penetrating power, but—because of their abundance and proximity to cell structures—are important in radiobiology. See *Radiation Hormesis,* page 2.

[4] Energies are in the range of 3 x 10^{20} electron-volts. For more information see *Scientific American,* January, 1999, page 32.

receive about 1,500 cosmic "hits" *per second,* each of which—because of the penetrating nature of all high-energy particles—collides with about 10,000 of the hundred-trillion cells in the adult human body. That's 15 million "cellular events" per second. If the quotation from Dr. Gofman at the beginning of this chapter is accurate, then we are indeed in a heap of trouble.

It is, by the way, the action of cosmogenic (a fancy scientific word for "from outer space") **neutrons** on atoms of atmospheric nitrogen that produces the carbon 14 used for radiometric dating.[5] Other neutron sources—accelerators, nuclear reactors, and bombs—have great potential for danger, as the lack of charge on the neutron allows it to penetrate some eight to ten feet of packed earth—about 50% farther than gamma radiation. Strictly speaking, neutrons are not ionizing radiation, since they have no electrical charge with which to influence the electrical affinity between protons and electrons. But they can smack into light-weight atoms such as hydrogen and cause them to become ionizing projectiles.

Finally, we have **X-rays,** which are typically produced when an energetic electron is stopped in its tracks. Just as with gamma rays, these can travel long distances and have the potential for doing harm to the body. During the past several decades, the energy—and therefore potential harm—of diagnostic medical X-rays has greatly decreased because of the increased sensitivity of the film and the detectors being used. Similarly, therapeutic X-ray equipment is designed to focus energy on smaller areas with less effect on healthy tissue. Sadly, an unwarranted fear of radiation causes many people who could be benefited by the use of X-ray diagnosis and therapy to

---

[5] Carbon 14 dating, developed in 1947 by W.F. Libby, is based on the fact that ^{14}C is continually produced by cosmic rays. When the high-energy ray collides with atoms in the atmosphere, free neutrons are produced which, when absorbed by a nitrogen (^{14}N) atom, cause it to eject a proton, thus converting it to ^{14}C. This radioisotope is taken in by plants and animals while they are alive but remains constant after death. By measuring the ^{14}C in comparison with its decay products, the approximate age of the fossil can be determined.

shun such treatment—and thereby become subjected to unnecessary *real* dangers.

A similar situation is found in the commercial/industrial environment where X-rays are subjected to such overprotective rules that their primary benefit—being able to detect flaws in welds and other material in order to protect human life—is rendered uneconomical. (No doubt there is also reluctance on the part of workers—who are victims of LNT theory fears—to use the equipment.)

All of the above forms of radiation are termed **ionizing radiation** because they have the ability to strip electrons from their orbits around nuclei, making the lone electron a negative ion and the "left-behind" proton a positive ion. Table 3 shows the electromagnetic spectrum illustrating the various kinds of ionizing and nonionizing radiation. For all practical purposes, ultra-violet radiation is not ionizing,[6] and it is the action of ionization that defines the beginning of the X-ray portion of the electro-magnetic spectrum.

The Concept of Half-Life

When an atom of a radioactive isotope decays, two things happen. First, energy is given off from the conversion of mass to energy according to Einstein's famous formula, $E = mc^2$. (The newly formed atom and any emitted particles are always lighter than the original atom—and it is this difference in mass that is converted to energy.) Simultaneously the original element is transmuted to an element with a lower atomic number. The secondary element is called the **daughter** (or **progeny**) of the first; it can be either a stable isotope or can itself be radioactive and go through a radioactive decay. Eventually, however, the original element decays to a stable form, and no more energy is given off.

---

[6] While UV radiation cannot ionize an atom, it can *dissociate* a molecule. For example, cosmic UV can smack into an O_2 molecule splitting it into two atomic oxygen atoms—which are very chemically active.

Table 3 The Electromagnetic Spectrum

<u>Non-Ionizing</u>

Radio waves (AM)—Long wavelength ~100 meters*

Shortwave Radio—Low frequency ~1 million Hz

Television VHF—Low energy ~10^{-9} electron volts

Television UHF

Radar

Microwaves (including ovens)

Infrared (heat) radiation

Red-Orange light

Green-Blue light

Ultraviolet A

Ultraviolet B

Ultraviolet C

<u>Ionizing</u>

Vacuum ultraviolet (absorbed by short path through air)

Low energy X-rays

Deep therapy X-rays—Short wavelength ~10^{-14} meters

Gamma rays (overlaps with X-rays)—High frequency ~10^{22} Hz

Cosmic photons—High energy ~100 million electron volts

* The ~ symbol indicates an approximate measure.

One can deduce from this that a radioactive element has a finite amount of energy to emit. Either it emits this energy very rapidly—in which case the radiation is intense and short-lived—or slowly, which would logically result in a relatively low radiation output. You can't have it both ways—a serious problem in nuclear medicine, as some of the intensely emitting therapeutic isotopes cannot be stored for more than a day.

Half-life is the time in which half the initial number of radioactive atoms decay.

If you stop to think about this phenomena, it's difficult not to have some kind of religious experience. Just think: In a tiny piece of (for example) uranium, one atom may have an internal "clock" that commands it to disintegrate in a second, while an adjacent atom in the same small sample will not decay for 13,500,000,000 years. How do they know when to "do their thing"? It's a problem that science may never solve.

Iodine 131 (used in thyroid diagnosis and ablation) has a half-life of about eight days. Thus if we started with a gram of ^{131}I, after eight days and fifty-seven minutes we would have only a half-gram with the other half having been transmuted to stable tellurium. In another eight days we would have only one-fourth. After eighty days—ten half-lives—there is less than $^1/_{1000}$ of the original specimen; beyond thirty half-lives, the isotope is considered to have disappeared. With its relatively short half life, ^{131}I is an intensely radioactive isotope.

Let's look for a moment at one of the most ubiquitous[8] radioactive isotopes around: ^{238}U, the primary uranium isotope making up 99.3% of the element's existence on Earth. It has a half-life of 4.5 billion years—approximately the same time estimated for the Earth's age. Uranium takes 207,000,000,000 times as long to decay as ^{131}I—with an inverse (longer time, less radiation) emission rate in approximately that proportion. Obviously it is a weak sister when it comes to being radioactive—which is fortunate for us or it would all be gone.

So, just in case I haven't made this clear, let me emphasize the following:

Short half-life = Intense emitter, but gone after a short time

Long half-life = Low activity and inherently not dangerous

---

[8] There are approximately 5,000 pounds of uranium in a volume of average soil one square mile by one foot deep.

Those who oppose nuclear technology want us to believe "Long half-life = Dangerous," but it's just not true.

Understanding the concept of **half-life** and its relationship to intensity makes one realize that Barry Commoner—when he invokes references to a "nuclear priesthood watching over wastes for thousands of years"—is either terribly ignorant himself or is hoping that we are.

Waste 'n' Time

Uh, oh. I'm afraid I've kind of painted myself into a corner here by minimizing the "problem" of nuclear wastes. If I give it short shrift, it will appear that I'm avoiding the subject. On the other hand, while the matter of nuclear wastes is somewhat afield from our general topic, there is a connection that might be of interest.

The only danger even attributed to nuclear wastes is that of causing cancer in future generations that are too stupid not to bite into a glassified chunk of power-plant waste. As we shall see, there is a threshold below which—even for these future glass munchers—there is no fear of increased cancer risk. But even if there weren't such a threshold, there are a number of issues regarding nuclear wastes that have been ignored in the media's misreporting of the subject that you should know about.

• More than 95% of the long half-life "waste" in nuclear fuel is not waste at all, but uranium and plutonium that may be reprocessed into fresh fuel assemblies. Most other industrialized nations do just this, as our government promised the utilities, but the Carter administration reneged on the agreement. (More about this later.)

• Among the "wastes" that anti-nuclear activists are eager to bury are valuable medical radionuclides that are produced at high cost in specialty reactors. As in the case of the reprocessable fuel, the baby is being thrown out with the bath water.

• The most sensible way to eliminate the unusable wastes from reprocessed fuel (which amount to about 1% of the fuel volume) is to dilute it a few millionfold and pour it down the drain, or to dump it into ocean abysses where there is no biological activity. Man's puny efforts at creating radionuclide wastes are dwarfed by the enormous amounts existing in nature. There are, for example, 36 billion curies of rubidium 87 and 380 billion curies of potassium 40 in the oceans, almost all of which will still be there when the few million curies of man's wastes have long since decayed to undetectable amounts.

Why then, you may ask, are there hundreds or thousands of government- (read "taxpayer-") supported scientists busy writing reports on Yucca Mountain? I suggest there may be three reasons: (1) they don't know—or, more than likely, don't care—that low-level radiation is not harmful; (2) it beats having to get a real job; or (3) grants to study the mating habits of the Zambian sweat bee have already been taken.

*   *   *   *   *

There's just no way to avoid the next subject, because, unless you get at least semi-comfortable with certain units of measurement, most of the book is not going to make much sense. We'll start by looking at a little shorthand "trick" used by lazy scientists and engineers.

One curie of radioactivity is a sizable amount. Many times a much smaller unit is needed especially when referring to amounts contained in milk, water supplies, and other common products. We could write this unit as 0.000000000001 curie, or 1×10^{-12} curie or spell it out as one-trillionth of a curie. But that's time consuming and a heck of a lot of trouble when you're writing it fifty times a day. The shorthand version for a trillionth of a curie is generally written as 1 pCi—or even 1 pC—with the "p" standing for pico and pCi referred to as a **picocurie**.

Similarly, 1 becquerel is a very tiny amount of activity amounting to one radioactive disintegration per second, while we often are interested in millions or billions of decays for a single gram of a

Table 4 International Standard (SI) Prefixes

Description	Factor	Prefix	Symbol
Quintillion	10^{18}	exa	E
Quadrillion	10^{15}	peta	P
Trillion	10^{12}	tera	T
Billion	10^{9}	giga	G
Million	10^{6}	mega	M
Thousand	10^{3}	kilo	k
Hundred	10^{2}	hecto	h
Ten	10^{1}	deka	da
Description	**Factor**	**Prefix**	**Symbol**
Tenth	10^{-1}	deci	d
Hundredth	10^{-2}	centi	c
Thousandth	10^{-3}	milli	m
Millionth	10^{-6}	micro	μ
Billionth	10^{-9}	nano	n
Trillionth	10^{-12}	pico	p
Quadrillionth	10^{-15}	femto	f
Quintillionth	10^{-18}	atto	a

radioactive isotope. So instead of a million Bq or 10^{6} Bq, it is written as MBq, with the *M* standing for mega.

Table 4 shows prefixes and their corresponding powers of ten. Since I find that use of so many prefixes makes comparisons difficult, I'll be limiting them to as few as possible. However, others will occur in quotations and in literature you might run across.

Well, we now know that radiation is caused by an atom suddenly going to pieces, but so far there is no clue as to why these particles are dangerous—if indeed they really are. So let's move on to some quantitative information about the effect of these atomic disintegrations.

Chapter 7
100 Picocuries—That's a Lot! (Or Is It?)

Since most Americans have no idea what danger might lurk in a glass of water with 200 picocuries per liter, we are at the mercy of those who might use this lack of knowledge to their political advantage.

IMAGINE SITTING IN a chair three feet away from a gram of an unknown radioactive metal, about the size of a penny, on the floor in front of you. Should you be concerned? I know I would be—at least until I knew more about what it was. Obviously we would be interested in what type of radiation was being emitted. If it were alpha or beta particles, there would be no problem as the 3 feet of air would stop any significant amount. But what if it were gamma rays? Then we would want to know just how "active" the source was—with the **activity** of a radioactive source being measured in the number of atoms that disintegrate every second.

Let's suppose our one gram of material is radium, specifically ^{226}Ra. Would you care to guess the number of disintegrations per second? A mere 37,000,000,000 (37 billion)! This, by the way, is the number of disintegrations defined as 1 **curie**, or 1 **Ci**, since the curie is defined as the activity of one gram of radium. You needn't run away, but you might not want to hang around. If it were one gram of cesium 134,[1] a quick exit would be advisable.

The curie, a United States (USA) unit, is still in common use but is gradually being replaced by the International Standard (SI) **becquerel** or **Bq**, which is defined as one disintegration per second. Obviously, then, 1 curie is equal to 37 billion Bq—not exactly the

---

[1] Cesium 134 is a gamma and beta emitter that has about fifteen times the activity of the Goian cesium 137, which is only a beta emitter.

Table 5 Specific Activities of Selected Elements			
Element	Curies	Becquerels	Half-Life
Thorium 232	.000000166	4,316	14.05 billion years
Uranium 238	.000000333	12,300	4.47 billion years
Potassium 40	.00000722	267,200	1.27 billion years
Radium 226	1	37 billion	1620 years
Strontium 90	139	5,143 billion	28.8 years
Cesium 134	1,290	47,900 billion	2.06 years
Iodine 131	124,000	4,588 trillion	8.04 days
Tellurium 133	113,000,000	4,200,000 trillion	12.4 minutes

easiest conversion constant to work with, especially when you have to go the other way: $1 \text{ Bq} = 2.7 \times 10^{-11} \text{ Ci} = 27 \text{ pCi}$.

A few elements of interest and their **specific activities**—that is, their activity per gram—are given in Table 5. Note that the half-life of the low activity ^{238}U is very long—4.5 *billion* years, while one-half the very active ^{131}I isotope is gone in 8.04 days. We would expect this, since there are a finite number of atoms in a gram of any substance, and if the rate of decay (i.e., the activity) is high, it will take less time for the substance to lose its radioactivity. This is verified by the very low relative activity of the **primordial radionuclides** such as thorium, uranium, and potassium, which have extremely long half-lives since these were presumably created at the same time as the Earth—estimated by most cosmologists as some 4.6 billion years ago. The shorter half-life isotopes—say a mere few million years or so—are long gone, although some are being replaced by decay products of the low activity elements.

When interested in relatively low-level radioactive material, the picocurie, or pCi (one-trillionth of a curie, remember?), is used. In Table 6, the activity is in pCi per liter and in Bq per liter.[2]

---

[2] You will also run across Bq per cubic meter (Bq/m3) in some radon studies. Multiply Bq/l by 1000.

Table 6 Specific Activities of Common Substances

Material	Picocuries/liter	Becquerels/liter
Normal air	2	.074
Typical radon level in Homes	3	.111
EPA limit: Ra-226 in drinking water	5	.185
Nuclear Power Plant Leak	15	.555
"Contaminated" milk at TMI*	22	.814
Rainwater**	360	13.3
Whiskey	1,200	44.4
Salad oil	4,900	181.5
Spa waters at Bad Gastein	16,200	599.
Drinking water in Maine***	53,700	1987.

*The increase in radioactive iodine in Harrisburg after the Three Mile Island "disaster" was 1/20 that caused by Chinese A-bomb tests in 1976. You remember how Jane Fonda and Ralph Nader protested those, don't you?

**Measured at Santa Fe, 5/11/86. (Probably atmospheric carbon 14 and wind-blown potassium 40 salts.)

***Based on an average of 226 samples. *Radiation Controversy*, Ralph Lapp, Reddy Communications, 1979.

Since most Americans have no idea what danger might lurk in a glass of water having 200 picocuries per liter, we are at the mercy of those who might use this lack of knowledge to their political advantage. Professor Petr Beckmann pointed out that activity in a well-publicized reactor leak at Indian Point power plant outside New York City was equivalent to that in a pint bottle of salad oil. Without this knowledge, an interested citizen would be led to believe (a) nuclear power was unreliable, and (b) such technology was a danger to life and limb—exactly what anti-technologists Nader, Commoner, Ehrlich, and their fellow primitivists would have us believe. Exactly the opposite of the truth.

You might want to bookmark this page, for easy reference to Table 6 as you read on.

In answer to the question posed in the chapter title, 100 picocuries is the approximate activity in a handful of average soil produced by the disintegration of potassium 40. (I always knew there was *something* dangerous about working out in the yard.)

Next we'll take a look at how the effect of ionizing radiation on the human body is measured.

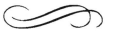

Chapter 8
Getting a Handle on Radiation Doses

 *How many atomic explosions in our cities would you accept before deciding that nuclear power is not safe—no complexities, just a number?*
—Ralph Nader, 1974

A SIGNIFICANT SOURCE OF confusion regarding the measurement of radiation parameters is the simultaneous use of two systems of units. As noted in chapter 7, "activity" is measured in curies in the USA system and Bequerels in the International System of units. A similar duality is found in the measurement of "doses" of radiation, as will be discussed in this chapter.

The question arises as to which units should be used in this book. Personally, I think in terms of the USA units and find that most people actively involved in radiation related disciplines in the United States do likewise. On the other hand, most scientific papers are written using the S.I. values—certainly all the recent ones on hormesis.

Since neither way will satisfy all readers, it will be the policy herein to use both in the next few chapters—generally the S.I. units followed by the USA units in parentheses unless a quotation or other source is expressed in the USA units... in which case the S.I. units are given parenthetically. Hopefully this repetition will get you accustomed to both systems of units and the relationship between them. Later chapters will use the same units as found in the source material. The plan is for you to become familiar with both by then and to make any necessary conversions in your head. (Or refer to Table 6 on page 51 or to Table 7, coming up on page 56, another good place for a bookmark.)

We will start with the more familiar (at least to me) USA units.

Measuring Radiation Doses

In the USA system of radiological measurements, there are three somewhat confusing units for measuring the *exposure to* and *doses of* radiation:

- the **roentgen**[1] (pronounced rent'-gen),
- the **rad**, and
- the **rem**.

To understand these you might imagine yourself on a sunny beach. The **roentgen** is analogous to the intensity of the sunlight striking the beach. The **rad** (radiation absorbed dose) corresponds to the amount of sunlight absorbed by your skin, while the **rem** (roentgen equivalent man) is comparable to the biological effect of the sunlight exposure. In the case of the rem, however, the difference in its effect is not due to your sunscreen, skin pigment, or hours spent in the tanning salon—but in the *type of radiation* being absorbed.

You may recall that the different *types* of radiation were either particles (alpha and beta rays, protons, neutrons) or high-energy photons similar to light (X- and gamma rays). Except for beta rays—which are electrons having some $1/1836$ the mass of protons or neutrons—the particles, because of their larger masses, have a more catastrophic effect when colliding with a cell in the body. For this reason the **quality** factor—usually designated as **Q**—is used to adjust the absorbed dose to its biological counterpart, the rem.

Mathematically, **rads x Q = rems**

Fortunately, most of the exposures we will be referring to in the study of hormesis are gamma and X-rays where Q is equal to one, allowing rads and rems to be used interchangeably. (Your radiologist, dental hygienist, and others working with X-rays will usually talk in terms of *rads* or *millirads*—but these are the same as *rems* and

---

[1] Wilhelm Roentgen (1845–1923) discovered an unknown emission (X-rays) from cathode ray tubes. It still happens today—that's how X-rays are made today. Incidentally, your TV screen is a cathode ray tube, and it emits many times the radiation we get from nuclear power plants. Somehow this fact escapes notice of the TV doomsayers.

millirems, because it is the X-ray source that produces the radiation.) There is one other term with which you should have at least a vague familiarity—Linear Energy Transfer or LET. Beta, gamma, and X-rays are considered low LET radiation, which means they have a Q of one. High LET particles can have Qs up to 400. A typical alpha particle has a Q of four.

The International Standard (SI) Units

In the International Standard measuring system, there is no equivalent for the roentgen—which is just as well as far as we're concerned because it is seldom used in relation to human exposure. The following relationships exist between the USA and SI units:

100 **rad** = 1 **gray** or **Gy**

and   100 **rem** = 1 **sievert** or **Sv**

One gray or sievert represents an *enormous* amount of radiation—about four times as much as a U.S. resident would normally receive in a 76-year lifetime. Smaller units, the **centigray, cGy,** and the **centisievert, cSv,** are more commonly used. These conveniently convert to USA units—

1 **cGy** = 1 **rad** = 1000 **millirad (mrad)**

and   1 **cSv** = 1 **rem** = 1000 **millirem (mrem)**.

If learning these measuring systems seems too complicated, try learning a few reference exposures and compare the value in question to these. Here are the ones I use, which then give me a feel for other values. After a while, they start all becoming second nature.

• **Sleeping with your spouse for a year—1 mrem** or .001 cSv (for the ambitious learner, .01 mSv). Since your spouse emits gamma rays; the rads, rems, cSv, and cGy are all the same. In almost all of the cases (except internal radium and plutonium) that we're going to be examining, this will be the case.

• **Background radiation in the United States—300 mrem** or 0.3 cSv. In the International System, the millisievert—one-tenth of the centisievert—is often used in this range. Our normal background dose in this unit is 3 mSv. Since a good portion of this radiation is from radon sources (an alpha emitter); rads, rems, Gy, and Sv are *not* interchangeable.

• **Radiation sickness—ensues at about 100,000 mrem,** or 100 rem, or 100 cSv, or 1 Sv. Because doses of this magnitude are usually low LET radiation, units of 100,000 mrad, 100 rads, 100 cGy, or 1 Gy may be used interchangeably. By the way, sickness results from an acute exposure of 1 Sv over a period of a couple of days or less. The same radiation over a longer exposure time gives no symptoms.

If you'll commit these three points to memory (or place a bookmark here), it will give you some frame of reference with which to compare other doses. Your bookmark will also give you easy access to Table 7, which gives some typical millirem and cSv values for other exposure situations.

Table 7 Selected Radiation Doses Per Year		
Source of Exposure	mrem	cSv
Nuclear plant within 50 miles	0.01	0.00001
Average Three Mile Island dose	0.1	0.0001
Color television	1.	0.001
One coast-to-coast jet flight/trip	5.	0.005
Border of nuclear power plant	5.	0.005
From food	25.	0.025
Cosmic radiation	27.	0.027
Building materials	34.	0.034
Your own blood (Potassium 40)	45.	0.045
On-site for duration, TMI accident	80.	0.080
One shoe X-ray (SXR)	175.	0.175
Grand Central Station	525.	0.525
Living on Colorado plateau	600.	0.6
Barium enema	800.	0.8
Max. permissible for nuclear worker	5,000.	5.
Radiation sickness (50% people)*	100,000.	100.
Death (50% of people)*	400,000.	400.
* acute exposure over a day or two		

Table 8   Acute Radiation Syndrome

	Subclinical Range 0–100 rads	Therapeutic Range 100–500 rads			Lethal Range 500+ rads	
		100–200	200–300	300–500	500–2000	2000+
Appropriate Action	None	Clinical Surveillance	Therapy Effective	Therapy Promising	Therapy Palliative (Comfort patient only)	
Incidence of Vomiting	None	100 rads: 5%, 200 rads: 50%	75%	75%	100%	100%
Delay Time	N/A	3 hours	2 hours	1 hour	3 min.	3 min.
Main Organs Affected	None	Blood Forming Tissue			Gastro-Intestinal Tract	Central Nervous System
Characteristic Signs	None	White Blood Cell Decrease	Fatigue; Infection; Erythema; Sterilzation; Loss of Hair above 300 rads; Hemorrhage		Diarrhea; Fever; Electrolyte Imbalance; Bleeding	Convulsion;Coma Loss of Muscle Control; Lethargy; Tremors
Critical Period	N/A	N/A	4–6 weeks		5–14 days	1–48 hrs
Post-Exposure Therapy	Assure of Safety	Blood Analysis; Assure of Safety	Blood Transfusion; Antibiotics	Possible Bone Marrow Transplant	Maintain Electrolyte Balance	Sedatives
Outlook	Excellent	Excellent	Good	Guarded	Hopeless	Hopeless
Convalescent Period	None	Several weeks	1–2 months	Long	N/A	N/A
Death Rate	None	None	0%–40%	40%–100%	90%–100%	100%
Death Within	N/A	N/A	2–4 weeks		2 weeks	2 Days
Cause of Death	N/A	N/A	Hemorrhage; Infection		Dehydration	Respiratory Failure; heart attack

Source: "Terrorism With Ionizing Radiation General Guidance: Pocket Guide," produced by the Employee Education System for the Office of Public Health and Environmental Hazards, Department of Veterans Affairs.

Some may think that certain data are emphasized in this and other chapters in an attempt to minimize the dangers of exposure to radiation. This is not at all true. I am trying to put the dangers *in perspective* and eliminate the Pavlovian negative response to even the very mention of the subject. Table 8 shows the accepted syndrome from short-term exposures. Please note that this table is in rems (not millirems) and can be mentally converted to centisieverts (cSvs) of the same numerical value. Radiation can obviously be very dangerous. But so can an unreasonable fear of radiation.

A Review

Before leaving dear old Hormesis U., here is a short review to see if you've got a handle on the curriculum. You should know…

- Elements are identified by the number of protons in the nucleus (atomic number).
- Isotopes of elements have different numbers of neutrons (n + p = atomic weight).
- Atoms of some isotopes are stable, while others are radioactive and, over time, will disintegrate (decay) into other elements of a lower atomic number.
- Alpha and beta particles have a short range (a few inches and a few feet respectively).
- Gamma rays and X-rays can penetrate several inches of steel or feet of concrete.
- The half-life of a radioactive isotope is the time it takes half of the original amount to decay; after thirty half-lives the original amount is considered to be gone.
- The longer the half-life, the lower the activity of an isotope.
- A curie is 37 billion becquerels.
- A pCi is a picocurie and is equal to one-trillionth (10^{-12}) of a curie.
- Absorbed doses of radiation are measured in rads or grays; 100 rads equals 1 gray.

- Biological doses are measured in rems or sieverts; 100 rems equal 1 sievert.
- The absorbed dose and the biological dose are the same for gamma and X-rays.
- A fatal acute dose is about 4 sieverts or 400 rems (50% fatalities in thirty days) when received in a relatively short time (a few days or less).
- Radiation sickness occurs at about 1 sievert or 100 rems (50% of those exposed over a short time).
- Doses below 1 sievert or 100 rems (100,000 millirems) have no immediate biologic effects but are generally thought to increase the risk of cancer in the future.

Thanks for your attendance at Hormesis U. No doubt you'll find the rest of the information on radiation hormesis much more understandable now than when you were a mere freshman. Oh, and be sure to send in your contribution to the Alumni Fund.

Chapter 9
A Very Short History of Radiation Hormesis

The extremely tall people on Niue Island (averaging height 6'6") receive 10 times more radiation from the soil than the world average.[1]

W HY, YOU MIGHT logically ask, was the hormesis phenomenon not discovered until some eighty years after Roentgen, Becquerel, and the Curies made their contributions to radiation science? Why was there not an earlier Professor Luckey?[2]

Actually there was of sorts, and he, oddly enough, was also a professor at the University of Missouri. In 1896, Professor W. Shrader inoculated guinea pigs with the diphtheria bacillus.[3] The group exposed to X-rays prior to inoculation survived; the unexposed cohort died within twenty-four hours. Shrader, in the same series of experiments, was apparently the first person to discover that "Roentgen Rays" could be used to kill germs.

During the early twentieth century, radiation was used for a variety of experimental therapies, but the doses were generally far above hormetic levels and may well have caused more harm than good. Patent medicines such as "Radithor" (more on this in chapter 24) were popular, with single doses having nearly a million times the daily radium intake allowed by current government regulators. Hundreds of thousands of vials of elixirs were consumed without any widespread harm occurring and with a sizable number of "miracle cures" being reported. Few controls, however, were em-

---

[1] Eugaster, Subradiation experiments concerning the concept of the natural radiation background, *Aerospace Medicine,* 35, 524, 1964.

[2] Professor Luckey is credited with coining with the term "Radiation Hormesis" from his 1981 book *Hormesis with Ionizing Radiation*

[3] Shrader, W. Experiments with X-rays upon germs. *Electrical Engineering,* 22, 170, 1896.

ployed to scientifically assess the actual worth of the treatments leaving one to believe that most of these "cures" may have been either the product of advertising hype or a placebo effect.

Medical research wasn't the big draw for world-class physicists. We might remember that in the early days of radiation experimentation important discoveries were being made almost daily, while health considerations—except, possibly, for the annoying, minor and superficial skin "beta burns"—were considered to be of no consequence. The doses of radiation these unprotected experimenters received are estimated to exceed by thousands of times the maximums under which today's nuclear industry workers are allowed to continue on the job.

Madame Curie, discoverer of both polonium and radium,[4] offers a good example of the "non-standards" of the day. It is anecdotal that whenever Marie Sklodowska[5] Curie walked into a room, electroscopes[6] immediately discharged. It is almost certain that she had an enormous lung burden of radium—the element she was extracting from uranium ore—which took quite a bit of patience, since there are only about 0.003 grams of radium per ton of ore. Madam Curie died almost certainly from the effects of long-

---

[4] In 1516, a silver lode was discovered in St. Joachim's Dale (Joachimsthal), which was—naturally—confiscated by the government of Count von Schlick. Coins minted from this mine were known as *Joachimsthalers,* which (for obvious reasons) came to be known as *thalers*—in English, dollars. It was from this mine that the Curies obtained pitchblende—an ore rich in uranium and its daughters, radium and polonium.

[5] In case you were curious why she named her first discovery for Poland.

[6] Gold is so malleable that it can be pressed into leaves less than $1/10,000$ of an inch thick. If you hang two pieces of leaf in an air-filled jar, with provision to charge both—you have an electroscope. Charging the leaves with the same polarity causes them to "push apart" and, because they are so light, the electrostatic "pushing" force exceeds the gravitational force that would cause them to "droop" into a vertical position. Such devices were used to assay the content of uranium ores—not from the non-penetrating alpha radiation of the uranium, but from the accumulated daughters of which the gamma ray emitting radium was a significant component. Air, when ionized, is a conductor that discharged the electroscope at a rate proportional to the amount of ionizing radiation present.

term and extremely high doses of radiation. Yet, at age sixty-six, she still exceeded by ten years the life expectancy of her day.

Later in the century, the subject of hormesis would have doubtlessly been trifling compared to other matters. From August 1939—when a letter from Albert Einstein was delivered to Franklin Roosevelt recommending the development of an atomic bomb— until the end of World War II, the focus of virtually the entire nuclear physics community became the Manhattan project. (This venture, equivalent in size to the total automotive industry at that time, is described in fascinating detail in *The Making of the Atomic Bomb*.)[7] Certainly the scientists were aware of potential dangers from radiation—especially the highly penetrating neutrons from "atomic piles"—but these risks were minimal, compared with the reality of thousands of deaths from the war every day. Concerns about low-level radiation—either harmful or beneficial—weren't even on the radar scope.

Interestingly, the only health physics experiment I've ever come across that occurred during the Manhattan project was indicative of radiation hormesis:

> In 1943, a group of [radiation scientists] on the Manhattan District Project were worried about the unknown toxicity of uranium. They grew a colony of rats in an atmosphere laden with sufficient uranium dust to kill them fast (the Manhattan Project didn't have time for fancy radiobiologists). As a control, a similar colony breathed clean air. After several months, nothing happened, but eventually the rats lived out their natural lifespan, with one surprise: the first health physics experiment demonstrated that rats who breathed uranium dust lived longer and were happier (i.e., had a better reproductive history) than normal rats. Not a tumor in the bunch.[8]

---

[7] Richard Rhodes, *The Making of the Atomic Bomb,* Simon & Schuster, New York, 1986.

[8] From a letter by Marshall Brucer, M.D. to *Time* magazine (from the files of Petr Beckmann).

During this period there are reports of relatively minor medical experimentation to determine the effect of ionizing radiation on the healing of wounds. The exposure levels, however, were high (1Gy or 100 rem)—suggesting its use as a bactericide. The availability of antibiotics in 1942, and the post-Hiroshima bombing concerns over high-level dangers, caused a loss of interest in research of this nature by the end of World War II.

After the war, the Japanese cities of Hiroshima and Nagasaki became laboratories for research on the effects of radiation on humans. But the focal point was on the high-dose subjects—in particular on their excess cancers and the possible mutational effects on children. When low-dose victims showed beneficial health effects, the data were ignored as being *anomalies* (a fancy scientific word for "it doesn't fit in with what we're expecting").

Luckey addresses this subject:

> Statistical analysis of observed data was missing in many reports of experiments involving low doses of ionizing radiation. Most of the reports simply indicated that an unexpected phenomenon had been observed, but the researchers failed to pursue it systematically.... Any unexpected result was rejected by the 95% rule: One experiment in each twenty was accepted as a variant. Closer inspection showed this was a consistent result; it usually occurred in the group exposed to the least radiation, the only one in the hormetic range. Hormetic data were ignored because they did not fit the models of the zero thesis.[9]

When someone *really* writes a history of radiation hormesis, the first "official" recognition of the phenomenon will go to the United Nations Scientific Committee on the Effects of Atomic Radiation (UNSCEAR) in a 1994 report "Adaptive Responses to Radiation in Cells and Organisms":

---

[9] *Radiation Hormesis*, p. 45.

Manifestations of the adaptation described in mammals after exposure to low doses of radiation include accelerated growth rate in the young, increase in reproductive ability, extended life-span, stimulatory effects on the immune system, and a lower than expected incidence of spontaneous tumours.

You might want to read that again.

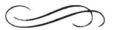

Chapter 10
A Day or So in the Life of a Cell

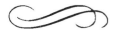 *Hormesis is not the action of radiation on a single isolated cell. But when a society of cells, such as an organ, is subjected to low-doses of radiation, protective action occurs.*

Hormesis, as discussed in chapter 4, is the stimulatory action of a low dose of an agent that would be poisonous in larger amounts. Two of the questions that come to mind in considering the radiation hormesis phenomenon are:

• How does radiation affect the body?
• What physiological processes could cause the hormetic effect?

Circle the Wagons

Many of us have heard that *the* problem with radiation stems from radioactive particles smashing into our cells, breaking up the genes, crushing chromosomes, and mutilating the DNA—thus causing a cell to grow wildly out of control, which we call a cancer. (If you didn't think that, there must be something wrong with you, because that's what most people think.) When visualizing such cellular violence, I suspect that most of us have some kind of model in mind. Mine was a golf ball-sized alpha particle crashing into a basketball-sized cell, trashing pencil-sized chromosomes—all relatively speaking, of course. In the worst case, there was the dreaded "double-strand break," whereby a golf ball would slice through both pencil-like DNA strands, leaving the cell with no template by which to repair the damage, as it normally would do. Call the oncologist.

When I learned a little more about what goes on in a cell during its workaday world—which we'll be getting to shortly—my model just wasn't making much sense. So I decided to look at the relative sizes of cells and their atomic enemies in hopes of being able to better imagine the processes that were going on during the collisions. It was surprising.

Let us consider an average animal cell, which is about 20 microns (millionths of a meter) in diameter, and hypothetically expand its cross-sectional area until it is the size of the field in Yankee stadium. And then let's take an alpha particle[1]—the shot put or bowling ball of the radioactive world—and enlarge it in the same proportion. What would you think? The alpha particle would be the size of a dump truck? A Volkswagen? (Too big.) A volleyball? A baseball? (Too big.) A pea? A B-B? (Too big.) The alpha particle, in relation to a Yankee-Stadium-sized cell, would be about 0.0003 inches in diameter—nearly the same as a human hair.

So what about damage inflicted by beta particles and gamma rays?

Beta rays are just speedy electrons, with $1/1836$ the mass of any one of the two protons and two neutrons making up an alpha particle. In terms of mass, the beta "particle" is a Ping-Pong ball compared with a 7.3-pound alpha-particle brick. When piercing our Yankee-Stadium-sized cell, the wound would be invisibly small, even with a magnifying glass. Say, maybe our cells aren't necessarily such wimpy victims after all.

Gamma rays and X-rays consist of **photons**, which, though devastating when loaded in Star Trek torpedoes, are "packets," or *quanta,* of energy that have essentially zero mass[2] and, therefore, zero size. Neither of these forms of ionizing radiation would make anything like a visible hole in our Yankee-Stadium-sized cell, but would pass though the cell walls like light though a dirty window.

---

[1] The nuclei of all atoms are surprisingly close to the same size. Uranium, while more than 200 times heavier, is only about three times as large as a hydrogen atom. The nuclei of both are on the order of one *barn* in cross-section, with the barn being 10^{-24} cm^2. (The term was occasioned when an early researcher remarked that a particular element's cross section looked as "wide as a barn.")

[2] If you really want to be picky, the photon can be considered to have mass because of the Einsteinian equivalency between mass and energy. But the photon exists in the form of energy and not mass as we know it.

With respect to the cell as a whole, radiation seems like mosquitoes attacking a circus tent, but once inside high-energy particles or rays can wreak havoc upon individual atoms and molecules that make up our cellular structure. Alpha particles, protons, and neutrons scatter whatever is in their path, using their mass energy to separate electrons from their parent nuclei. Beta rays whiz though a thin layer of cells, knocking other electrons out of their orbits until their rather limited energy is expended. Gamma and X-rays act similarly, but with a vengeance proportional to their energies and inversely proportional to their wavelengths.[3] Usually they still have plenty of spunk after zipping through our bodies stripping some 10,000 electrons out of their formerly contented orbits in the process.

Whenever an electron and its former nucleus partner (the proton) are separated, the atom is **ionized**—with the electron being a negative ion and the electron-starved nucleus being a positive ion. While we've been taught that the dreaded "double-strand breaks" are the main problem, the cell has a way to take care of these, which we'll get to soon. The primary cause of cellular damage from ionizing radiation is, by gosh—**ionization**.

When an electron is stripped away from a water molecule— and these make up some 99% of a cell's cytoplasm (the stuff inside the cell's membrane but outside the nucleus)—the normally placid water molecule turns into the Mr. Hyde of the cellular world. Good old H_2O is converted into strange entities like hydroxyl radicals (OH^-), which will fight anybody or anything to hook up with another electron. These are the feared "free radicals," which are the targets of heroic "anti-oxidants" seen in all health food magazines.

Just as I was completely off base on my concept of relative sizes of atoms and cells, I also had misconceptions about cell activities. I assumed they lived a rather boring life interrupted occasionally by

---

[3] Light, which is part of the same electromagnetic spectrum as both X- and gamma rays, behaves similarly. Long wavelength infrared light—otherwise known as radiant heat—has very little energy compared to short wavelength ultraviolet light…which can "ultraviolate" you on the beach if you don't use sunblock.

having to split into two cells. From time to time, however, a bullet of radiation might penetrate the cell, causing it to marshal its defenses—for a battle that would often be lost—and an almost inevitable cancer would result. It's not a totally irrational model if you've been led to believe that all radiation is hazardous. But it's not even close to being true.

Just in case your cellular biology is a bit rusty, let's look for a moment at a typical animal cell. It is surrounded by a membrane that somehow knows what substances to let into and out of the cell. Inside the cell—besides cytoplasm—is the nucleus, which contains the *nucleoli* and the *chromosomes*. (The *nucleoli* busy themselves making the RNA and protein.) Chromosomes are long, threadlike bodies consisting of a single DNA molecule coiled tightly inside. In humans, the molecule is thought to be around sixteen inches long, but so thin that it cannot be resolved with an electron microscope.[4] Only about 10% of the DNA is active in providing instructions for the cell's growth, functioning, and reproduction. The remainder (essentially archives of the cell's history) is sometimes referred to as "junk DNA."

As far as being a peaceful environment, the cell makes a beehive appear laid-back. There are roughly 200,000 DNA repairs *every day* in *every cell* with some 30,000 unrepaired breaks existing at any given time. About 2% of these are the dreaded-double-strand breaks.

So *most* of this is caused by radiation? Hardly.

Normal oxidative damage—arising from thermal instability, replication, and free-radicals spawned by normal cell activities—is the overwhelming cause of DNA alterations. For the average U.S. citizen receiving a background dose of 0.3 cSv (300 mrem), the radiation-produced DNA breaks number six per cell *per year*. Even a fatal dose of 1000 cGy (1,000,000 mrad) produces only 20,000 breaks per cell—a mere 0.03% of the normally occurring 70 million alterations per year.

---

[4] In the Yankee Stadium example, the DNA molecule would be about 4,000 miles long but possibly too thin to be seen with the unaided eye.

It would appear from this that radiation should have little effect on us one way or the other. Insofar as directly causing cancer, that is indeed what the evidence in future chapters will show. As Theodore Rockwell[5] puts it,

> It is the repair and removal process (or lack of it) that kills us. Like other toxins, high-level radiation degrades those processes, but low-level actually stimulates them.

As anyone with the least familiarity with radiation knows, high levels of radiation are dangerous and can kill you (Table 8). The low-level effects may be new to you, but they are real and are arguably far more important for society than the almost infinitesimally rare occurrences of high-level exposures.

Hormesis Mechanisms

Every second the average person in the United States is "hit" by 15,000 particles of ionizing radiation, mostly from background sources. (The 1,500 "hits" mentioned earlier were only from cosmic sources.) Why does a relatively small increase in this exposure have a positive effect on the health of individuals? That physiological changes occur is unquestionable: it has been known for almost a century that low doses of radiation increase the production of lymphocytes (white blood cells). Other changes observed to occur are:

- Increased number of immune system helper T cells
- Decreased number of immune system suppressor T cells
- Increased activity of the p53 protein[6]

---

[5] Ted Rockwell, Sc.D. is the former technical director of U.S. Naval Reactors. The American Nuclear Society's Lifetime Contribution Award has been named the Rockwell Award in his honor.

[6] A protein that reputedly decreases the incidence of many cancers.

• Increased free-radical scavenger activity (while radiation causes the creation of free radicals, it simultaneously produces much more of the remedy than of the problem).

The above, among others, are considered to be part of the cell's defensive system against chemical and radiation insults. Interestingly, *high* doses of radiation have a "reverse effect" on these very same cellular activities.

In the previous quotation from Dr. Rockwell, it was noted that a poor job in the cellular repair and removal business is what causes us potentially fatal problems. The body just doesn't do well with a bunch of sick, dying, or dead cells hanging around. An interesting discovery resulting from the hormesis research led by Dr. Sohei Kondo[7] was that low-dose radiation increased **apoptosis**—often referred to as altruistic cell suicide. By this process damaged cells were absorbed without necrosis (a fancy scientific way of saying the cellular bodies were carted off before becoming offensive) and, at the same time, healthy cell replacement was stimulated.

In considering what hormesis *is,* we should also be aware of what it *isn't.* It is *not* the action of radiation on a single isolated cell. In experiments involving single cells *in vitro,*[8] they behave as the LNT theorists would predict: the more radiation, the less vitality.[9] But when a *society of cells,* such as those making up an organ or an organism, is subjected to a relatively low dose of ionizing radiation, protective action (homeostasis) occurs, and the effect can be quite dramatic, as will be shown in the chapters on evidence.

One final analogy: we are aware that introducing the cowpox virus into our body causes the immune system to gear up and

---

[7] Dr. Kondo is professor emeritus of Biology at Osaka University, and senior researcher at the Atomic Energy Research Institute, Kinki University, Osaka, Japan.

[8] Literally, in glass—although almost all "glass" dishes these days are actually plastic.

[9] Critics of hormesis often point out isolated cell experiments as proof against the phenomenon.

produce antibodies that also happen to be effective against small-pox. What isn't commonly known, however, is that inoculation against one disease increases the body's resistance to others. A 1986 English study showed a decrease in death from malignant disease for all who were inoculated, as children, for any one of eight diseases. Children inoculated against measles, for example, had a better chance to survive diphtheria or whooping cough, even while lacking those specific inoculations.

Similarly, low doses of radiation "inoculate" the body to the negative effects of future high doses—while at the same time appear to have positive effects in increasing general immune competency. Those who would like to learn more about radiobiological and hormetic effects should find the references in chapter 15 to be interesting. They allude to the Japanese research on the subject, which is well ahead of that being done in the United States.

Chapter 11
You Can Run, But You Can't Hide

 *If an increase in low-level background radiation caused any problems, decades of anecdotal evidence would have made Denver a ghost town.*

No ONE ESCAPES radiation. As mentioned earlier, the average person receives 15,000 "hits" *each second*, while a medical X-ray may easily score some 100 billion cellular incidents.[1] Those who say that "it takes only one gamma ray to cause cancer" may be technically correct, but they neglect to mention a small statistical detail: The odds against any particular gamma ray causing cancer in an affected cell are 1 out of 30,000,000,000,000,000. (That's 30 quadrillion, or 30×10^{15}, to one.) Besides, hormesis evidence indicates that the gamma ray of concern is more likely to *prevent* cancer than to cause it.

Before defining the units used to measure radiation exposure, you may recall we used the SXR (shoe X-ray) as a yardstick to compare the dangers posed by various radiation sources. As you may have guessed, the SXR is not exactly a reference unit recognized by the scientific community. A more convenient benchmark would be the average background exposure that we receive from the various natural and man-made sources. But, as we'll see, this "natural background" value varies by a factor of a hundred or so in different locales on planet Earth—almost all of which is the fault of nature, not man. Still, it would be desirable to reference other levels of radiation to *some* normal amount; so we'll arbitrarily use, as a definition of "natural background," the exposure to the average U.S. citizen—previously mentioned to be 300 mrem from natural sources and 63 mrem from man-made (mostly medical) origins.

---

[1] Risk of Nuclear Power, by Bernard L. Cohen, University of Pittsburgh professor. You can read the entire article at http://www.physics.isu.edu/radinf/np-risk.htm

Until the twentieth century, the average background dose of radiation for a human being had continually decreased over our species's existence because of the slow decay of the primordial radionuclides such as thorium 232, uranium 238, and potassium 40. So what happened during the 1900s that turned the curve upward?

Most people would answer (a) fallout from atom/hydrogen bomb testing and (b) nuclear power plants. Nice try, but no cigar. Bomb tests did inject huge amounts of highly radioactive materials into the atmosphere, where most decayed to safe levels within ten days of testing. Other longer-half-life isotopes[2] from fallout caused a temporary worldwide increase of background radiation in the neighborhood of 1% to 4% depending mainly on location. Today it amounts to less than $1/1000$ of the average background level. As mentioned, there has been only a single "fall-out fatality" from atom/hydrogen bomb testing, which occurred on the misnamed *Lucky Dragon*. While antinuclear statistics have killed off many (theoretical) thousands in their quest for an atomic scapegoat, our inaccurate friends have been unable to directly attribute any other death or injury to radiation from fallout, except as a statistical article-of-faith based on the discredited LNT and "collective dose" theories.

Nuclear power plants, on the other hand, have known emissions of radioactive products such as xenon (a non-reactive "noble" gas), but these are so low in practice as to be immeasurable. It is calculated that the average U.S. resident receives a dose considerably less than 1 mrem from all nuclear power plants combined—again, as with fallout, about $1/1000$ of the normal background radiation. For those truly troubled by potential radiation exposure, it is not necessary to avoid being in the vicinity of power plants, but you might want to stay away from the U.S. Capitol building and Grand Central Station, both of which emit considerably more radiation than would be legal for any U.S. *nuclear* power plant to emit.

---

[2] The one of primary concern being strontium 90 with a half-life of twenty-nine years and a propensity to replace calcium in bones.

So where did the increase come from?

If we are to believe a report from the National Academy of Sciences Committee on the Biological Effect of Ionizing Radiation (BEIR IV), most of the increase came from weather-stripping, storm doors, and polyethylene wrapping of new homes. Not that any of these products was unusually radioactive, but because they made houses "tight," thus causing radon gas, which bubbles up from decaying radionuclides in the soil, to be trapped in the living areas. This, they calculate, amounts to 200 mrem per year—unless, as we shall see, you are fortunate enough to get more.

The second largest component of the increase is from X-rays and nuclear medicine. The averages used for medically related exposures are somewhat misleading, however, since they range from a 1-mrem dental X-ray to about 100,000 mrem (100 cGy) for a thyroid ablation.[3] In other words, most people fall well below the combined 53 mrem medical dose, while a few have relatively massive doses. As the evidence section will show, even these huge doses of X-rays or medical radioisotopes produce no measurable increase in cancer—and indeed are seen to have a hormetic effect in those cases where low-level effects were investigated.

Finally, about 10 mrem comes from consumer products such as smoke detectors, television receivers, and tritium watch dials. *None* comes from the process of food irradiation for a very simple reason: The process physically can not make the food radioactive. Does having an X-ray make *you* radioactive? Same thing.

Table 9 gives a breakdown of sources in the United States, according to the BEIR committee. Obviously, for most of us, our largest dose of radiation comes from natural sources. The exposures from "man-made" sources are almost entirely voluntary. If you don't want to have a dental X-ray, then don't. If your doctor

---

[3] In 1979, the University of Michigan outfitted the husband of a woman undergoing radioactive iodine thyroid diagnosis with a dosimeter. They found that *he* received a dose of 2,500 mrem(!) during their vacation—which would no doubt cause the EPA to forbid them to sleep together.

Table 9
Sources of Average Annual Radiation for a U.S. Citizen

Natural Sources	mrem/yr	cSv/yr	% Total
Radon	200	0.2	55
Cosmic*	27	0.027	8
Terrestrial	28	0.028	8
Internal	39	0.039	11
Total Natural	300	0.3	82
Man-Made Sources			
Medical X-rays	39	0.039	11
Nuclear medicine	14	0.014	4
Consumer goods	10	0.010	3
Nuclear power	< 1**	< 0.001	–
Fallout	< 1	< 0.001	–
Total Man-Made	63	0.063	18
TOTAL	363	0.363	100

* Doubles for every 6000 feet in altitude.

** (The symbol "<" means "less than")

Source: Department of Energy Report YMP-0337 from BEIR IV. Available in its entirety at http://www.ocrwm.doe.gov/factsheets/pdf/ymp0337rev1.pdf

wants to check your thyroid function using iodine 131, tell him, "No thanks, I'll just feel awful for the rest of my life." If you don't want a smoke detector in your home, then don't buy one; burn your family up if that's your preference. Don't watch television or use a computer terminal.

But to avoid the natural background radiation, you need to take some pretty serious steps. Moving to Antarctica or living underwater in a nuclear submarine are your best bets. Or you could also move from high-background-radiation Colorado (with a *low* age-adjusted cancer death rate) to the low-background-radiation southeastern and eastern coastal states (with *high* age-adjusted cancer death rates). Then again, you might move out of your high-radon-exposure home in the Reading Prong of Pennsylvania to an area with a lower radon dose rate... but with a higher lung cancer toll.

You're not going to do any of these things. Why? Because if an increase in low-level background radiation caused any problems, we would see evidence—in the form of dead bodies. Decades of anecdotal evidence would have made Denver a ghost town, and Leadville, Colorado—the city with the highest altitude, and therefore the most cosmic radiation—would have only monuments to its former short-lived citizens. But the only people who think that there is any such danger are the regulators, anti-nuclear activists, "environmentalists," and government scientists—who cling to the Linear No-Threshold (LNT) Hypothesis. We will be discussing this concept as applied to ionizing radiation, but since our government is so concerned about the doses we receive in this county, let's see what the situation would be if we lived with the background radiation experienced by fellow human beings who live in places *outside* the United States.

Remember, the average background radiation in the United States is 300 mrem (.3 cGy) plus an average of 63 mrem, primarily from medical sources. And remember that the radiation rules-makers are out to regulate public exposures down to a single mrem (.001 cGy); they intend to put a limit on public exposures at 100 mrem (0.1 cGy).

Breaking News!! EPA Restricts Foreign Travel Because of Dangerous Radiation Levels[4]

The highest background radiation levels I could find are in China, India, Brazil, and Iran (more on this in chapter 17). All these countries have deposits of monazite—a black sand often found on beaches and in rare earth deposits—in which the principle radioisotopes are from the decay of thorium 232 and radium 226.

The 80,000 people of Kerala, India, receive up to 1,300 mrem (1.3 cSv or about three-and-a-half times our background exposure)

---

[4] Well, not yet really... but give them a little time.

Table 10   Background Radiation in Various Locations with Comparisons*

Case/Place	cGy/yr	mrem/ year	Ratio to U.S. average
EPA level of concern	.001	1	.003
Limit nearby nuclear power plant	.005	5	.016
Proposed EPA maximum (all sources)	.100	100	.3
U.S. Average background	.300	300	1.0
Chernobyl forced resettlement**	.500	500	1.7
Colorado plateau	.600	600	2.0
Kerala, India	1.3	1,300	4.3
Gerais, Brazil	2.3	2,300	7.7
Hormesis optimum (Luckey)	10.0	10,000	33.3
Guarapari Beach, Brazil	26.3	26,300	87.6
Ramasari, Iran (average)	48.0	48,000	132.

* Adapted from "Radiation Hormesis for Health" by T.D. Luckey, *Health Physics Newsletter,* June 1995.

** In areas where the natural background plus the Chernobyl contribution exceeded this limit, 200,000 people were forcibly resettled.

per year and have been recognized for their healthfulness compared with neighboring states. The 10,000 citizens of Guarapari, Brazil, and the vacationers that flock to their beaches to bury themselves in the black sand absorb 0.03 mGy (3 mrem) per hour—the equivalent of 26,280 mrem (2.6 cSv or about eighty-seven times our background) per year.[5] Meanwhile in Ramasari, Iran, the 2,000 inhabitants and their ancestors have lived for centuries being exposed up to 48,000 mrem (48 cSv or 132 times the U.S. average) and "sur-

---

[5] It is illegal to take the sand, but it has been done for centuries by tourists who have heard of its benefits and keep it under their beds. By so doing they receive little additional "through skin" radiation, but are exposed to continuing sources of breathable radon.

vived" to tell about it…in fact they keep on surviving to the point that our regulators are wearing out their fingernails from scratching their LNT—and collective dose—heads. (Actually, they just engage in politically correct science: *ignore those data that are inconvenient.*)

Chernobyl—Symbol of Unconcerned Totalitarianism

One can hardly compare the Chernobyl fire in the Ukraine to the alleged "Three Mile Island disaster" in Harrisburg, Pennsylvania. Thirty-one firemen and plant workers were killed in the former, while the only victims at TMI were from media-caused anxiety. Volumes have been written by analysts on the mistakes made at both power plants. But Chernobyl, with its graphite reactor designed to produce weapons-grade plutonium as well as electricity—and with no containment building—cannot even be compared with the pressurized water reactor (PWR) at TMI in which the nuclear reaction is stopped by the laws of physics when there is a loss of coolant water. Of course that hasn't stopped the anti-nuclear, anti-technologists from trying. But perhaps the strangest story out of Chernobyl was that the Soviet hierarchy, who had strongly supported the anti-nuclear activists in the United States, were apparently led to believe their own propaganda about radiation dangers.

The accident at Chernobyl provided both good and bad news for anti-nuclear activists. For decades, they had been attempting to come up with some reasonable way that radioactive products from nuclear power plants could be spread over the countryside. The best they'd been able to come up for U.S. power plants went like this:

(a) A loss-of-coolant accident occurs, and the emergency core cooling systems fail to operate, leading to a meltdown of the fuel assemblies inside the reactor.

(b) Although the nuclear reaction stops when the coolant is lost (the water acts as a moderator to slow down the neutrons so they can be captured and allow the reaction to continue), there is still heat generated from the decay of the "daughters" of the reaction. This is supposedly so intense that it melts through six inches of steel in the reactor vessel, and continues through many feet of high-strength, reinforced concrete.

(c) But it can't stop there. The molten mass must then continue to melt through perhaps a few hundred feet of earth until reaching an aquifer. There the steam generated causes "blow holes" to develop, and the steam carries the radioactive products back to the surface. (Hold on, we're almost there.)

(d) The weather must cooperate with a gentle breeze blowing toward a populated area. (Too much wind and our "cloud" dissipates; under calm conditions, the product settles to the earth at the facility and is taken care of there.)

But the graphite fire at Chernobyl provided an actual way that about *90 million curies* of radioactive material could be efficiently spread around the county side. Yes, the anti-nukes got their dream of a large scale nuclear disaster—which had been becoming more and more difficult to conjure up, given the fact that Three Mile Island showed that the uncovered fuel elements couldn't even melt through the reactor vessel.

But there was bad news for them also. There weren't any bodies in the streets. Aside from those who died on-site, mostly firemen who expired from burns with possibly complications from radiation, there is no sign of a cancer epidemic or any other chronic problem.

Oh, sorry, there's one. The governments involved are going broke (brok*er*?) from the payments they are making to victims. Victims? Didn't I just say there weren't any victims? Yes, but I meant from the radiation. The victims as defined by the governments involved are those who were traumatized by *fear* of radiation or from the trauma of being evicted from their homes and forced into refugee camps.

Of the radionuclides escaping from the burning graphite reactor at Chernobyl, the one of most concern was cesium 137. A gamma emitter with a half-life of thirty years, this reactor product settled to Earth over much of Europe. Yes sir, it did. But nobody seemed to notice it settled right on top of soil that already contained naturally occurring radioisotopes, such as ^{238}U, ^{232}Th, and ^{40}K. In

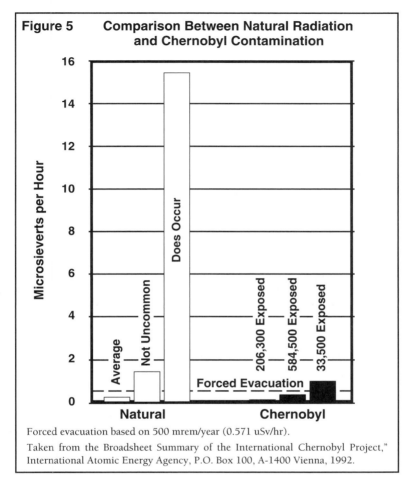

Figure 5   Comparison Between Natural Radiation and Chernobyl Contamination

Forced evacuation based on 500 mrem/year (0.571 uSv/hr).

Taken from the Broadsheet Summary of the International Chernobyl Project," International Atomic Energy Agency, P.O. Box 100, A-1400 Vienna, 1992.

a mistaken spirit of humanitarianism, the Soviet Army evacuated its citizens when the dose from the Earth exceeded 0.5 cGy (500 mrad) per year.[6] They apparently didn't notice they were already sitting on "highly radioactive" dirt. Figure 5 shows the Chernobyl contamination relative to naturally occurring radiation. Is it any wonder that the "Project Team's Main Recommendations" included the following?

---

[6] One of the purposes of this book is to show how some authorities—even nuclear officials—have no connection with reality and, indeed, make recommendations and rules that cause great harm. This example shows nationality is no barrier.

Measures with less impact on traditional agriculture should be investigated; better public information is needed, *particularly on doses and risks,* and studies of the acceptability to people of living in contaminated areas. [Emphasis added.]

Table 11 Chernobyl Cs 137 Burden in Various Areas vs. Natural Background	
Location	Range (Bq/m^2)
European Cs 137 contamination outside former USSR	20,000 to 23,000
Cs 137 contamination inside former USSR	40,000 to 5,000,000
Natural radionuclides in soil of above areas	177,000 to 6,500,000

Source: Table 2 in 1997 statement by U.N. Scientific Committee on the Effects of Atomic Radiation (UNSCEAR) member Zbigniew Jaworowski.

Table 11 gives another look at the Cs 137 "fallout" and the natural radionuclides in the top 10 cm (about four inches) of soil in several locations around Chernobyl. Note the range of natural soil radiation. Wouldn't you think that someone would have noticed a variation in the detrimental effects of natural radiation when some areas had thirty-six times the soil radioisotopes of others—*if indeed there were any detrimental effects?* Wouldn't you think one area would be known as *Cancervania*—because of regular affliction of the populace from radiation, while another area would go by *Vitalia,* because of superior health derived from a dearth of radiation exposure? But we don't see Europe having such disparities in cancer or other immune disorders on the basis of location, do we?

Well, actually we do: the health resorts are almost always located on springs with a high radon content.

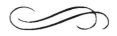

Chapter 12
Radon: Scourge or Blessing for Mankind?

 *Government was tightening industrial radioactive emission standards to ridiculously low levels, while demanding that homeowners modify their homes to the point where radon doses to the average citizen were hundreds of times greater than the levels dictated to nuclear workers.*

R ADON IS THE HEAVIEST of the "noble gases," so named because it—like its cousins neon, argon, krypton, and xenon—does not react with other elements to form compounds. It is radon's "nobility" that minimizes its effects on the body, since it is mostly a transient that is breathed in and then expelled without any chemical reaction taking place. When radon decays in the body, however, it spawns a series of short half-life progeny that are not only chemically reactive with tissue, but are—as we would suspect from their half-lives—also highly radioactive.[1]

Hazard to Miners?

For years, radon has been thought to be a hazard for miners, and a special confusing unit of activity—the Working Level (WL)—was derived to measure the danger.[2] Recently, however, as evi-

---

[1] When uranium decays (which isn't very often with a half-life of 4.5 billion years), the products of the decay go through four more stages (taking a couple of million years) until radium is formed. With a half-life of 1,600 years, radium 226 decays into radon gas with a half-life of 3.8 days. The daughters of radon are polonium 218, lead 214, bismuth 214, polonium 214—and a couple of others. The aforementioned have very short half-lives and are therefore highly radioactive.

[2] One WL is the activity of air containing 100 pCi (3.7 Bq) of radon in equilibrium with its daughters (which, by the way, virtually never happens in the real world) per liter of air. For an approximation, a Working Level Month (WLM) is equivalent to a one-time whole body dose of about 300 mrem (.3cGy).

dence of radiation hormesis has emerged, the jury is back out to deliberate a reconsideration of radon's guilt. It is now recognized that other carcinogens—in particular, the particulates suspended in the air of all mines and, more recently, the fumes from diesel engines—were present, but never considered. Radon was *assumed* to be the carcinogenic culprit, a theory that appears now to be based on flimsy circumstantial and anecdotal evidence.

A related re-evaluation of lung cancer in the Joachimsthal[3] mining community noted that victims were invariably "pensioners," i.e., *miners* (not their unexposed, above-ground cohorts) who had made it to a retirement age, which was about ten years *longer than their life expectancy*. One might easily speculate that the cancer was caused by microscopic dust lodged in the lungs and the miners' long lives a beneficial product of radon gas.[4] There has also been a piece of the puzzle right under our noses.

Radon gives its dose of mixed radiation primarily to the bronchial epithelium (fancy scientific words for "windpipe"), hence one would expect cancers caused by radon to be concentrated in this area. *Au contraire!* The miners' cancers are deep in the lungs,[5] similar to the cancers caused by the South African *amphibole*-type asbestos,[6] used in ships because of its resistance to brine, acids, and oils. It is difficult *not* to see the parallel between non-degradable asbestos fibers in the lungs and non-soluble silica particulates found in most mining environments.

---

[3] A famous mine in Czechoslovakia—as you already know if you read footnotes, as you ought to be doing.

[4] One of Europe's most famous health spas is *Bad Gastein* near Salzburg, Austria, which advertises "air with the highest radon content in Europe." The activity of its water is noted in Table 6.

[5] Nobel Laureate Rosalyn Yalow, Radiation and Society, *Interdisciplinary Science Reviews*, 16, 4, 1991.

[6] Not to be confused with the common, domestic serpentine type of asbestos, which has not been shown to cause disease.

Home Is Where the Radiation Is

From Table 11, radon is apparently the dominant source of background radiation. As pointed out earlier, it has not always been considered to be such, as residential radon seems not to have existed until December 1984, when a nuclear worker set off radiation alarms on his way *into* the Pennsylvania Limerick power plant. A subsequent investigation showed that the residential radon level in the Reading Prong area of Pennsylvania and New Jersey exceeded the level found in many mines. Always quick with a horror story, the EPA "found" this new "danger" to millions of citizens and gleefully reported that as many as 20,000 lung cancer deaths in the United States are caused by residential radon. Perhaps someone at the EPA should have been reading a certain $36 per year newsletter.

Petr Beckmann was well aware of this noble gas situation, as evidenced by 106 different mentions of radon in his newsletter *Access to Energy*[7] from September 1979 through June 1992. Professor Beckman was wise enough not to condemn the radon levels out of hand, but he took the bureaucrats to task for their double standard: One hand of government was tightening industrial radioactive emission standards to ridiculously low levels, while the other hand was encouraging/demanding that homeowners modify their homes to the point where radon doses to the average citizen were hundreds—if not thousands—of times greater than the levels dictated to nuclear workers. Here is an example from the November 1983 edition of his newsletter—prior to the EPA's "discovery" of residential radon:

> Although radon exposures of the public are regularly hundreds and even thousands of times higher than from nuclear power operations, that alone may not be cause for alarm. Our purpose here is not to

---

[7] Now edited by Dr. Arthur Robinson, President and Research Professor, Oregon Institute of Science and Medicine, Box 1250, Cave Junction, OR 97523. Back issues, twenty-one-year CD-ROM, and index available.

Gasteiner Heilstollen

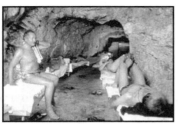

In the Healing Gallery in Gastein deep down in the Radhaus Mountain, there is a worldwide unique healing climate to be found: Because of the air, which contains radon and temperatures of 37 to 41.5 degrees, and a relatively high humidity of between 70 and 100%, your body will refill itself naturally with vitality and strength. Muscles and joints relax as the mountain gives out new energy.

The Healing Gallery in Gastein is the most effective treatment method in Gastein and is probably the most effective natural healing method for treating rheumatic illnesses.

The Natural Healing Power:
- High Radon content (up to 4.5 NanoCurie per litre of air in the Gallery)
- Damp warmth (air temperature ranges from 37–41.5°C a relatively high air humidity of 70/100%).
- Speleotherapy Conditions (completely pure, dust free, allergy free, and practically bacteria free air, healing aerosol, negative ions)

(above copy taken from http://www.gastein.com/en-gesundheit-heilstollen.shtml)

OR

EPA Recommends:

- If you are buying a home or selling your home, have it tested for radon.
- For new homes, ask if radon resistant construction feature(s) have been used.
- Fix the home if the radon level is 4 picocuries per liter pCi/L) or higher.
- Radon levels less than 4 pCi/L still pose a risk, and in many cases may be reduced.
- Take steps to prevent device interference when conducting a radon test.

(above copy taken from www.epa.gov/iaq/radon/pubs/hmbyguid.html)

WHOM TO BELIEVE? Spas in the Bad Gastein area of Austria have been known for their health benefits since Roman times—while the U.S. EPA didn't discover radon as a *threat* until 1984. Note that the level in the "healing gallery" is *1,000 times* the "fix it" level of the EPA.

scare readers with the dangers of radon, but to point out the inconsistency of the media and of the politicians bent on pleasing them.

When it came to radon, one might ask about the government's myopia for so many years. Well, one might also remember that during this period we were having one of our regularly scheduled energy crises and were being urged to seal up our residences and commercial buildings. (Anyone born before 1960 should surely remember Carter's "thermostat cops.") Without ventilation, the heavy gas, almost eight times heavier than air, seeps into basements or lower floors with additional amounts coming from unvented or poorly vented natural-gas heaters. There appears to have been a contest between which "crisis" was more important—energy or radiation. *Energy shortage* was first out of the gate, but it's *radiation* coming down the homestretch.

Bane of the EPA

In 1990, the first of Bernard Cohen's studies was published showing that *higher* household radon levels were associated with *lower* lung cancer rates. The wealth of evidence rocked the scientific community, most of whom had never bothered to question the Linear No-Threshold model. They were to be even further "rocked" by his even more comprehensive report in 1995. He is still [2005] evaluating even the most unlikely confounding possibilities that might discredit his highly significant findings. As a seeker of scientific truth, Cohen is working diligently to prove himself wrong.

The evidence chapters of this book contain many references to radon, including a whole chapter on Cohen's study (chapter 20). It might be a good idea for you to read them prior to spending big bucks for a government-approved, radon-reducing heat exchanger, which allows circulation without appreciably changing the temperature of the room air.

A Parting Shot in the Radon Controversy

Since it affects only air passageways and the lungs, radon and its progeny do not really give us a "whole body dose" like most of the other radiation sources that provide our background dose. Its contribution of 55% of our natural background is therefore given as an "equivalent whole body dose" calculated from the 2,400 mrem dose given yearly to the bronchial epithelium times an "effective dose equivalent factor" of 0.08. This calculated dose of about 200 mrem (.2 cGy) is tied to the LNT and might make sense if the linear theory were true—which it is not. In my opinion, the BEIR data on radon and its effects are worse than meaningless. They are unscientific, fraudulent, *and* meaningless.

Chapter 13
Rummaging Through the Stacks

Where the radiation level is greater,
cancer risk is invariably less.[1]

PRESENTING THE EVIDENCE of radiation hormesis has been the most daunting problem faced in writing this book; there is just too much of it. Luckey had more than 2,000 citations in his two books,[2] and he estimates that this was about half of the data available in 1990. In the fifteen years since then, other researchers have become involved, and their research compounds the problem of "too much" evidence. Until of late there had been only a very few experiments *designed* to address the radiation hormesis hypothesis, and most of these involved non-vertebrates.[3] The data available—which are the backbone of the argument I'm putting forth[4]—are generally one of the following types:

- Animal tests designed to find adverse effects of *high levels* of ionizing radiation but which happened to take measurements in the low-dose area in the course of the experiment;[5]

---

[1] Nambi and Soman. Further observations on environmental radiation and cancer in India, *Health Physics,* submitted in 1990, unpublished.

[2] *Hormesis With Ionizing Radiation,* CRC Press, Boca Raton, 1980; and *Radiation Hormesis,* CRC Press, Boca Raton, 1991.

[3] Even more rare are *subambient* (i.e., less than normal background) radiation experiments, which should show a degradation of biologic function when the target microbes are shielded from cosmic and other background sources. Two such experiments are described in *Radiaion Hormesis,* pp. 211–23.

[4] While I have absolutely no reason to distrust the recent test reports that attest to the hormesis phenomenon, there is something very satisfying about examining data taken without any conceivable bias toward "the reverse effect." If there were any bias it was to ignore that which didn't fit the curve.

[5] According to Luckey, much of the low-dose data—which showed negative correlation of the dose-response relationship—was either ignored, omitted, or simply deemed too unimportant to report.

- Japanese bombing survivors who were within a known distance of A-bomb detonations and whose exposures could be calculated;[6]
- Statistical evidence on workers in nuclear power plants and weapons manufacturing facilities, and
- Populations that live in various areas with background radiation up to eighty times the U.S. average.

It would be wonderful if there were carefully controlled experimental data on humans for all diseases over the complete radiation dosage range. To optimize the hormesis effect, it would be marvelous to have double-blind studies over long periods of time, with carefully controlled exposures and rates. But we don't have these things.

Coming Mother...

This is where evaluation of the evidence by an informed and sensible citizenry comes into play. As matters stand now, we have a "nanny" government that dictates what is good for us and what is not. The government regulators who determine the "rules" usually do so in a manner that will make them popular with those they think are important—it's a process called *politics*. And almost every "rule" they make has a single stated purpose: to protect us from something, someone, or ourselves. If our FDA had been around in Edward Jenner's 1796 England, how many people would have died from smallpox waiting for a bureaucracy to approve vaccinations?

With regard to our subject matter, a presentation by a Canadian regulatory official[7] offers a case in point. The radiation expo-

---

[6] There is considerable controversy about exposures, particularly in Hiroshima, with many researchers believing the data analysis understates the radiation dosage. One problem is related to some data still not being available to investigators—even after more than fifty years!

[7] At the 1998 Ottawa Conference on Low-Dose Radiation.

sure regulators are well aware of the eventual demise of the LNT and the strong evidence that low-level radiation is beneficial. These are not "bad" or conspiratorial activists who want to destroy Canada. But will they consider relaxing the already miniscule limits (5 mSv or 500 mrem) for public exposure to radiation? Will they adopt a policy raising limits for hormesis studies? *Absolutely not!* They intend to lower the limit even further to 1 mSv (100 mrem)!

Because of a clear and present danger? Not at all. It is because of political pressure from the "all-radiation-is-dangerous" crowd and eagerness on the part of the regulators to avoid a confrontation with the politically powerful "green lobby." What, pray tell, would it take for the regulators to change their minds and look at the evidence? (I copied this one down verbatim.) They will not consider changing "without the other worldwide regulatory agencies agreeing to adopt it [the less stringent regulations]."

Let's see now, if country A won't change until B, C, and D have changed; and country B won't change until A, C, and D have changed…gee, it doesn't seem like there's going to be a whole lot of changing going on.

Battling the Bureaucracy

I'd suggest that the only way to change country A's regulators would be for the citizens of A to understand the evidence and know the evidence proves the regulators are wrong; that their regulations are costing lives, not saving them; that the tax money of the citizens is being wasted on nonsensical programs to reduce radiation levels that are already insignificant; and that people and industries are being denied the benefits of nuclear technology because bureaucrats feel a responsibility to "enforce official policy" rather than question, observe, and reason.

So, I submit, it is up to *us* to look at the evidence—of which the following is just a small fraction—and then, with reason and eloquence, persuade our political leaders to lead. Failing that, we should work to throw the blackguards out, and help elect those who *will* listen to reason—and not to the anti-technologists who would return us to the days of manure, a boring subsistence, and back-breaking labor.

In Luckey's *Radiation Hormesis,* the source of much of the evidence to be offered in the upcoming chapters, the subject matter was arranged in terms of parameters that were being observed, e.g., fertility, growth rate, immunity, mortality, cancer risk, life span. Subjects of the studies ranged from bacteria to fish eggs, to mice, to beagles, to humans—with each interspersed within the observed parameters. The information presented is technical, quite detailed, and frankly—because I tend to faint when reading italicized Latin words of more than two syllables—can be a bit difficult to understand. But that's what we engineers were put on Earth for: to attempt conversion of scientists' idea into something *normal* people can fathom.

For this reason I've concentrated on, and am limiting the data to, studies on mice and men. Mice, because the experiments are with statistically significant numbers of specimens bred to minimize genetic differences—and men (women, too) because of a hunch that readers will be interested in that particular species. Additional details on these and related subjects can be found on the Radiation, Science, and Health website at http://cnts.wpi.edu/rsh.

Upcoming chapters have the following content:

Chapter 14	Data from mice experiments concerning responses, such as longevity and various cancer mortalities, to a wide range of exposures
Chapter 15	Observations and data from A-bomb survivors
Chapter 16	Radiation effects on workers in nuclear power plants and nuclear-weapons facilities
Chapter 17	Effects of different levels of background radiation on residents in different geographical areas

Hopefully, one or more of these topics will be helpful in your evaluation of the experimental basis of hormesis—or, as United Nations Scientific Committee on the Effects of Atomic Radiation (UNSCEAR) puts it—"the adaptive response to radiation in cells and organisms."

Chapter 14
Who's the Leader of the Gang...

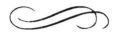 *Irradiation of the pregnant animals—and the foetuses in utero caused an astonishing decrease of the mortality rate of the infected baby mice.*[1]

As a rule, I don't think much of animal experiments. No, I'm not a member of People for the Ethical Treatment of Animals (PETA); in fact, I think many test animals (that would have never existed were it not for testing requirements) have it a whole lot better than their cousins who live in the wild. Can you think of anything worse than being a mouse that is in the process of being swallowed whole by a snake? And besides not having to be constantly on the lookout for snakes, cats, and hawks, some of these test critters have a pretty active social life—especially those involved in reproductive studies.

My problem with much of the animal testing is similar to the problem I have with the LNT—it is based on extrapolation with no consideration of a possible (and likely) threshold. For example, cancer researchers will load up some rat—which has been bred for a propensity to have tumors—with the human equivalent of two boxcars per day of an artificial sweetener, and then declare the substance to be a human carcinogen when a few tumors appear. No consideration is given to the possibility that there is a threshold, above which the rat's resistance is overwhelmed, but below which there is no effect.

Fortunately, mouse experiments related to disproving the LNT and demonstrating hormesis are not in this category. A single

---

[1] Mayr and Paulas, Unexpected effects of a whole body irradiation on the mortality rate of baby mice after an experimental infection with the vesicular stomatitis virus (VSV), *Zentralbl. Veterinaermed,* 36, 577, 1989.

datum point on the accompanying graphs is often the average of hundreds of mouse lifetimes, and the curves subsequently drawn lie within the range of these experimental data so that no extrapolation is necessary. Besides most of the tested mice should be happy campers, since ionizing radiation in the hormesis range generally promotes health and longevity.

This chapter will look into the effects of low-level (and a few not so low-level) X-rays and gamma radiation on the mice. Most of it is related to cancer, since, as we are aware, this disease is commonly associated with radiation and is, in fact, *the major* detrimental effect of exposure. Other topics include growth rate, life span, radio-resistance (which all parents of teenagers should have), and one inexplicable effect of radiation received *by the parents* of the test mice.

In all the following studies, exposures (rads/Gy) and doses (rems/Sv) are equal, since only gamma and X-ray radiation are involved.

Growth Rate of Irradiated Mice

In a 1954 study by E. Lorenz et al.[2] on the "effects of long-continued total body gamma irradiation on mice, guinea pigs, and rabbits," it was found that the growth rate of mice increased in proportion to the exposure, up to the level of 1.0 cGy (1,000 mrad) *per day.* Above this point, as shown in Figure 6, the growth rate decreased, until it was the same as the control group at approximately 7.5 cGy per day. Irradiation, which lasted eight hours per day, commenced one month after birth and continued until death. This study did not, however, examine the question of the relative longevity of the mice involved—a subject taken up later in this chapter.

The size advantage (considered "healthy" in mice, though probably not popular in Minnie's ballerina class) continued into late maturity—about 100 weeks.

---

[2] Lorenz, Egon, et al. Effects of long-continued total body gamma irradiation on mice, Guinea pigs and rabbits, in *Biological Effects of External X and Gamma Radiation,* Vol. 1, Zirkle, R. E., ed., McGraw-Hill, New York, 1954.

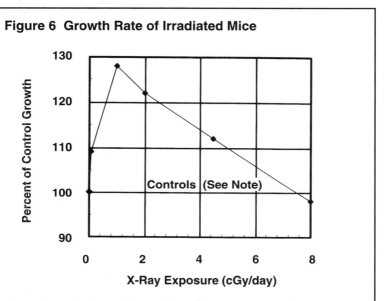

Figure 6 Growth Rate of Irradiated Mice

Note: "Control" or "Controls" refers to a group of unexposed animals often as large as the entire exposed cohort. The average behavior of this group is the norm to which all other groups are compared.

Source: Lorenz, E., Jacobson, L.O., Heston, W.E., Shimkkin, M., Eschenbrenner, A.B., Deringer, M.K., Doniger, J., and Schweistal, R., Effects of long-continued total body gamma irradiation on mice, Guinea pigs, and rabbits. III. Effects on life span, weight, blood picture and carcinogenesis and role of intensity of radiation. In *Biological Effects of External X and Gamma Radiation,* Vol. 1, Zirkle, R. E., ed., McGraw-Hill, New York, 1954.

If we consider the background level to be the U.S. average of 0.3 cSv or 300 mrem per year (about 1 mrem per day),[3] then the fastest-growing rodents received about 1,000 times their normal background radiation—hardly in keeping with the LNT—which would predict unhealthiness at any level above background. It strongly suggests beneficial radiation effects are at work.

---

[3] The dose (expressed in units of energy per mass) is independent of the size of the recipient.

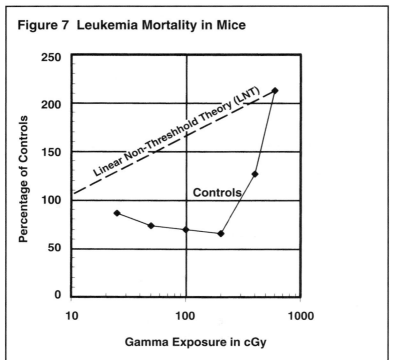

Figure 7 Leukemia Mortality in Mice

Source: Maisin, J.R., Wambersie, A., Gerber, G.B., Mattelin, G., Lambiet-Collier, M., and Guelette, J., Life shortening and disease incidence in C57BL mice after single and fractionated gamma and high energy neutron exposure. *Radiation Research,* 113, 300, 1988.

Effects of Radiation on Cancer—Leukemia Mortality

Of the myriad varieties of cancer, leukemia is most often considered to be associated with exposure to ionizing radiation, so we'll look at it, first, in an experiment involving 1,000 young adult mice per group (about 12,000 mice in all), which were exposed to a single dose of gamma radiation from 20 to 600 cGy at the rate of 300 cGy (300 rad) per minute. (Ouch.) This experiment was directed by J.R. Maisin and reported in *Radiation Research,* 113, 300, 1988 (see Figure 7). To realize just how far apart the Linear No-Threshold theory and the hormesis model are from one another, the LNT predicts a 60% *increase* in leukemia at an exposure of 200 cGy, while the actual data show a 35% *decrease.* One can argue all day the beauty of the LNT and how it is a terrific standard for regulatory control; but these data show that it just isn't true when compared to experiment.

Effects of Radiation on Pituitary Cancer Mortality

In 1979, R.L. Ullrich et al. compared the pituitary cancer mortality rate of 400 female mice exposed to single doses of 10, 25, 50, and 100 cGy.[4] The normal mortality from this cancer in the control mice was 6.6%—a value that was set as the 100% or control level on Figure 8.

As shown, pituitary cancer mortality was decreased nearly 20% at an exposure of 25 cGy, which was similar to results for ovarian cancer (20% decrease), mammary cancer (46% decrease), and

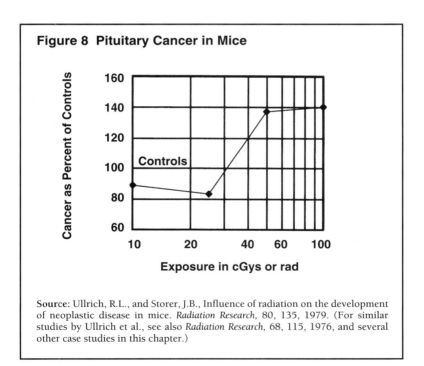

Figure 8 Pituitary Cancer in Mice

Source: Ullrich, R.L., and Storer, J.B., Influence of radiation on the development of neoplastic disease in mice. *Radiation Research,* 80, 135, 1979. (For similar studies by Ullrich et al., see also *Radiation Research,* 68, 115, 1976, and several other case studies in this chapter.)

[4] Ullrich, R.L. et al. Influence of radiation on the development of neoplastic disease in mice. *Radiation Research,* 80, 135, 1979.

uterine cancer (13% decrease). Needless to say, these are not the kind (or even the direction) of results predicted by the LNT.

Effects of Radiation on Cancer in Mice—Lung Cancer Mortality

There are three studies that address the effects of ionizing radiation on lung cancer mortality in mice. The most recent of these was a 1997 experiment by Y. Hosoi and K. Sakamoto[5] in which mice were injected with artificial metastases (a fancy medical term for cancer cells) and then irradiated with gamma rays up to 100 cGy (100,000 mrad). Data showed the lowest cancer rate in a range between 15 and 40 cGy, with the minimum being 41% of controls at 15 cGy.

The Hosoi–Sakamoto study demonstrated another tenet of the hormesis theory, however, which most other experimenters have neglected to investigate—namely, that hormesis is a property of the organism and *not* its individual cells. When tumor cells that had been irradiated with 10 to 50 cGy gamma rays *in vitro* were injected in the mice, there was no difference from the controls—indicating that the suppression affects the mouse, not tumor cells. Unfortunately, the study involved only 200–250 mice (perhaps they are scarce in Japan?) and lacks the statistical significance I would like to see for compelling evidence.

Both of the other lung cancer experiments were performed by Ullich et al., whom we have seen laboring earlier with mouse pituitaries; and both experiments involved several thousand mice. His 1977 investigation,[6] which showed a minimum lung cancer mortality in the area of 100 cSv, was repeated in 1979.[7] This time, instead of only two data points, six were examined from 10 to 300

---

[5] Suppression of spontaneous and artificial tumors by low dose total body irradiation in mice. In *Low Doses of Ionizing Radiation: Biological Effects and Regulatory Control*, International Atomic Energy Agency, TECDOC-976, Vienna, 1997.

[6] Ullrich, R.L., et al. Neutron carcinogenesis. Dose and dose-rate effects in BALB.C mice. *Radiation Research*, 72, 487, 1977.

[7] Ullrich, R.L., et al. Influence of irradiation on the development of neoplastic disease in mice. *Radiation Research*, 80, 135, 1979.

cSv. As shown in Figure 9, the minimum appeared around 25 cSv in the 1979 data but was still significantly lower than controls even at the 100 cSv level.

At the risk of sounding repetitive, it is evident that the LNT is completely inadequate to explain this phenomenon, while the hormesis theory predicts just such a occurrence.

Effects of Radiation on the Life Span of Mice

Surely if ionizing radiation has beneficial effects on growth rate and the immune system competence of mice, as evidenced by a decreased susceptibility to cancer, it ought to have a positive effect on life span. As several studies demonstrate, this is indeed the case.

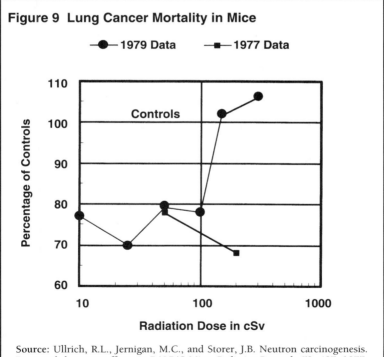

Figure 9 Lung Cancer Mortality in Mice

Source: Ullrich, R.L., Jernigan, M.C., and Storer, J.B. Neutron carcinogenesis. Dose and dose-rate effects in BALB/C Mice, *Radiation Research*, 72, 487, 1977. Also Ullrich, R.L., and Storer, J.B. Influence of irradiation on the development of neoplastic disease in mice. I. Reticular tissue tumors. II. Solid tumor. III. Dose-rate effects. *Radiation Research*, 80, 135, 1979.

A 1983 investigation[8] by J.B. Storer was cited by Luckey as an example of how hormesis effects are often overlooked by researchers who are expecting a bio-negative response from radiation.[9] The authors ignored a peaking of longevity between 5 and 10 cGy, hopefully not in any attempt to be fraudulent or unethical, but probably because it would have appeared anomalous in terms of the LNT.

It is an earlier study[10]—which most certainly gave unintended results—that is of considerable interest to hormesis researchers. Life spans of mice—90 in a control group, and 90 to 120 in four exposed groups—are plotted in Figure 10 on the basis of daily

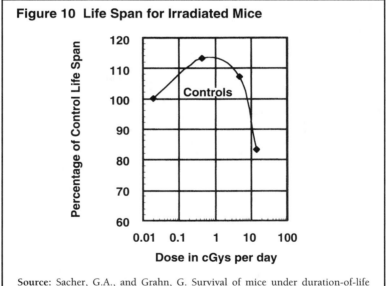

Figure 10 Life Span for Irradiated Mice

Source: Sacher, G.A., and Grahn, G. Survival of mice under duration-of-life exposure to gamma rays. I. The dosage-survival relation and lethality function. *Journal of the National Cancer Institute,* 32, 277, 1964; also *ANL Report 6971,* 1964, p 94.

---

[8] Storer, J.B., et al. Life shortening [sic] in Balb/C mice following brief protracted, and fractionated exposures to neutrons. *Radiation Research,* 96, 396, 1983.

[9] *Radiation Hormesis,* 1981, pp 46, 50.

[10] Sacher, G.A. and Grahn, G. Survival of mice under duration-of-life exposure to gamma rays. *Journal of the National Cancer Institute,* 32, 277, 1964.

exposures to cobalt-60 gamma radiation. Exposures, which began 100 days after birth, were continued until the death of the specimen.

Anti-nuclear activists, "animal rightists," and "popular wisdom" would predict dire consequences for test animals subjected to such huge doses of radiation *every day of their lives*. But this study offers substantial evidence that mice receiving 1,000 times their normal background dose had the longest life spans.[11] You might recall that, in the earlier discussion of growth rate, the optimum was also 1,000 times normal background.

Parlez-Vous Radiation?

Using lower exposures than the Lorenz and Sacher experiments, a study by French researchers[12] documented the effect on 900 mice— 300 controls, 300 receiving a chronic gamma ray dose at the rate of 7 cGy/year, and 300 exposed similarly to 14 cGy/year.[13] Quoting from the abstracted results of the *Gerontology* article,

> The life span, after the beginning of the experiment, determined by the survival time of 50% of each population, is increased in irradiated mice: 549 in controls, 673 days in both irradiated groups. The differences are significant between the control and the irradiation mice. Differences between mice irradiated with 7 or 14 cGy are not significant.

So what did the researchers conclude?

> These results confirm the possibility of a non-harmful effect (hormesis) of ionizing radiation. They demonstrate that the para-

---

[11] It is my understanding that similar results were reported by a researcher named Searle in 1964, but I have not been able to obtain any more information.

[12] Caratero, A., Courtade, M., Bonnet, L., Planel, H., and Caratero, C. Effect of a continuous gamma irradiation at a very low dose on the life span of mice. *Gerontology*, 44, 272–76, 1998.

[13] These exposures are twenty-three to forty-six times the U.S. background level.

digm, which states that low-dose effects can be predicted [by] high-dose effects, cannot be systematically applied in radiation biology in general and gerontology in particular.

Doesn't sound like there's much vacillation here, does it?

Before moving on to evidence on two-footed subjects, there are a couple of other unusual mouse studies that merit consideration.

Radio-Resistance in Mice Previously Exposed to Hormetic Levels

We are aware that inoculations strengthen the immune system by mildly stressing it and causing antibodies to arise that fight any further intrusion of a similar type invader. In effect, vaccinations are examples of hormesis: *Small doses of poison are stimulatory.* The poison in this case is a virus, not an inorganic toxin. Hans Seyle (chapter 4) doesn't care what it is. As long as it stresses the host organism, it starts an alarm reaction that stimulates a defense mechanism.

If radiation hormesis is a valid concept, we might expect small doses of radiation to ward off the bio-negative effects of higher doses—obviously not through the creation of antibodies but by some currently unknown mechanism. Figure 11 illustrates just such a phenomenon.

In this 1990 experiment by M. Yonezawa et al.,[14] mice were irradiated with a low dose of X-rays (50 cGy or 50,000 mrad) two weeks before a second potentially lethal dose of 740 cGy (740,000 mrad). The survival rates of the irradiated group were compared with the unexposed controls. There isn't much question as to which mouse group I'd want to line up with on "inoculation day."

Table 8 (in chapter 8) shows the dose-response for humans is similar to that which Yonezawa finds for mice—at 700 rem, we're both dead or close to it. Would humans have a similar radio-

---

[14] Yonezawa, M., et al. Acquired radioresistance after low-dose x-irradiation in mice. *Journal of Radiation Research*, 31, 1990.

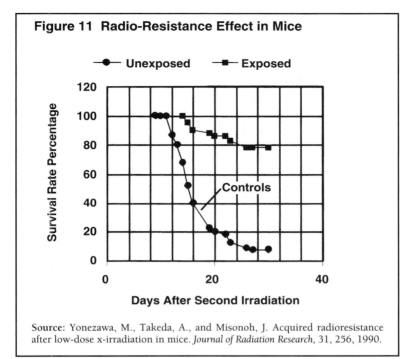

Figure 11 Radio-Resistance Effect in Mice

Source: Yonezawa, M., Takeda, A., and Misonoh, J. Acquired radioresistance after low-dose x-irradiation in mice. *Journal of Radiation Research,* 31, 256, 1990.

resistance response? We don't know and aren't likely to until the knee-jerk reaction to anything nuclear is abated by scrapping the LNT. If I were a nuclear worker—involved in changing fuel elements where high-level (but so far, nonfatal) accidents have occurred, or an astronaut potentially subjected to a cosmic radiation barrage, or perhaps a soldier with the potential for high-level exposure from a neutron bomb, I think I'd want someone to look into the radio-resistance phenomenon who wasn't committed to the LNT hypothesis and likely to state at the outset, "All radiation is harmful—and it's our job to keep you from having any."

Very Strange—But I Don't Make the Data; I Just Report Them

The next figure is about mice that were not subjected to radiation but who had fathers that had been exposed prior to becoming a mouse-parent. (Yes, I realize this may be sounding a little like Psychic Hotline.) Figure 12 shows the life span of unexposed mice, who were fathered by mice (naturally) that had received 30, 70, 100, or 150 cGy of X-rays at sixteen weeks of age. (Irradiating the mother mice had no effect on the life span of their progeny.)

How do *I* explain such a phenomenon? I haven't the foggiest idea…and I don't think anyone else does either. But if there were a possibility I could add 20%–40% to the life span of my child by exposing myself to 100 cGy of radiation, that wouldn't be much of a decision. It is questions like these that we should be setting the stage for future generations to answer. Instead we are planning how to waste some $1 trillion cleaning up "nuclear dumps" that are less radioactive than the natural soil in many parts of our world.

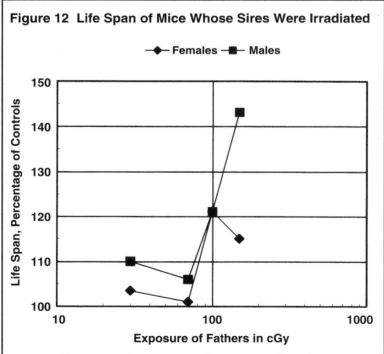

Figure 12 Life Span of Mice Whose Sires Were Irradiated

Source: Spalding, J.F., Brooks, M., and McWilliams, P. Some effects of X irradiation in successive generations on an inbred and hybred [sic] population of mice. *Genetics,* 50 (Supplement), 1179, 1964. Also in *Effects of Ionizing Radiation in Reproduction,* Carlson, W.D. and Gassner, F.X., editors. Pergamon Press, London, 1963

You're probably tiring of mousy data, and I said we'd get on to humans after a couple more reports on rodent experiments. We'll just breeze right though these and let you practice your mental conversion from cGys to rads or cSvs to mrems (they are all the same for the radiation in all these citations).

• "The effect of neutron exposure [3.2 cGy–6.3 cGy] upon the combined sexes showed low doses *decreased* the natural incidence of all tumors."[15] [Emphasis added.]

• Mice exposed to 150,000 mrem at five and twelve days following infection with "friend [sic] virus" recovered while all of the controls died within forty days.[16]

• "[Studies on mice] in the dose range 0–3 Gy by two independent research groups at Oak Ridge and at Casaccio near Rome leads, for gamma radiation and X-rays, to a statistically significant *decrease of the cancer rate at low doses* and therefore to biphasic relationships for tumors of the reticular tissue, for several solid tumors, as well as for cancer as a whole."[17] [Emphasis in the original]

• "Male mice exposed to acute doses of 2 Gy for 82 successive generations showed no abnormal offspring; this acute dose is equivalent to 50 times background radiation for humans from the time of the Roman Empire to present."[18]

---

[15] Meweissen, D.J, and Rust, J.H. Reticuloendotheial neoplasms in C57 black mice after fast neutron irradiation at low doses. *US Atomic Energy Commission Conference 740930*, Oak Ridge, 1976.

[16] Shen, R.N., Hornback, N.D., Lu, I., Chan, L.T., Drahms, Z., and Droxmeyer, H.E.,. Low dose total body irradiation; a potent antiviral agent *in vivo*. *International Journal of Radiation Oncology and Biological Physics*, 10, 185, 1989.

[17] Weber, K. Biphasic dose-effect relationships in experimental studies of radiation cancer in animals. [English summary.] *Strahlenbiologie und Strahlenshutz*, Hannover. October 1996. IRPA, Progress in Radiation Protection.

[18] Spaulding, J.F., Brooks, M., and McWilliams, P. Some effects of X irradiation in successive generations on an inbred and hybred [sic] populaiton of mice. *Genetics*, 50(Suppl.), 1179, 1964. Also in *Effects of ionizing radiation in reproduction*, Carlson, W.D. and Gassner, R.X., eds., Pergamon Press, London, 1963.

• "Urinary testosterone of chronically irradiated mice, 5,000 to 10,000 mrem of X-rays per day, was increased 264% above controls."[19] [Look out, Viagra.]

• Of the offspring of 124 male mice exposed to 276,000 mrem of X-rays and 124 control mice, 20 of 3,990 pups from exposed males were stillborn, as compared to 45 of 3,418 control pups.[20]

• In an experiment involving 3,505 autopsied mice with acute exposures of 18 cGy or more, the age-specific lymphocytic lymphoma rate was 16% of controls for 36 cGy exposures and 3% for those exposed to 18 cGy.[21]

• Radio-resistance—the resistance to high levels of radiation exposure—in mice was enhanced by previous exposure to lower levels of X-rays. Survival of mice exposed to 700,000 mrem increased from 10% in the control group, to 25%, 50%, and 82% for exposures to 120,000 mrem at one, two, and three weeks of age, respectively.[22]

• Mice that had been exposed—from weaning through breeding—to 1 cGy/day had shorter generation times and higher birth rates than unexposed controls.[23] [A later experiment on "deer mice" by the same researchers gave similar results.]

• " For newborn mice exposed to 180 rad at 0.07 R/day, the life span was significantly longer than it was for controls. At all dose

---

[19] Liu, S.Z. Effects of low dose ionizing radiation on defense and adaptive mechanisms. *Conference on High Background Area Research,* Taishan, Nov 1988; *China Medical Journal,* 102, 750, 1989.

[20] Luning, K. Studies of irradiated mouse populations. *Hereditas,* 46m 668, 1960.

[21] Meweissen, D.J, Rust, J.H., Harem, J., and Clement, M.J. Assessment of dose-response relationships in carcinogenesis following low radiation dosage. In *Late effects of ionizing radiation.* International Atomic Energy Agency, Vienna, 1978, 291.

[22] Kochanski, W., et al. Immunologic analysis of the condition of increased resistance of organisms exposed to ionizing radiation. *Medical Radiology,* (Moscow) 1, 43, 1956. [Hmm, why would they have been interested in such a subject?]

[23] French, N.R. and Kaaz, H.W. The intrinsic rate of increase of irradiated *Peromyscus* in the laboratory. *Ecology,* 49, 1172, 1968.

levels the 2-month age group lived significantly longer than did the median controls."[24]

• "Male AKR mice were irradiated with 5 cGy three times a week or 15 cGy two times a week for 11 weeks from age 40 weeks. The incidence of thymic lymphoma was 80.6% in sham-irradiated mice [controls], 67.5% in mice irradiated with 5 cGy three times a week, and 48.6% in mice irradiated with 15 cGy twice a week."[25]

*   *   *   *   *

Gee, I could go on about mice for hours...unfortunately I wouldn't have any readers. So let's move on to the evidence that alerted so many people to the truth of Dr. Luckey's claim of radiation hormesis: the Japanese survivors and their stubborn refusal to die on the LNT schedule.

---

[24] Patterson, H. Wade, editor of the *Health Physics Journal,* elucidating experimental data by Spalding, J.F., Thomas, R.G., and Tiejen, G.L. in *Life Span of C57 Mice as Influenced by Radiation Dose, Dose Rate, and Age at Exposure,* Report No. UC-48; LA-9528, Los Alamos National Laboratory, 1982.

[25] Ishii, K. and Watanabe, M. Participation of gap-junctional cell communication on the adaptive response in human-cells induced by low-dose of X-rays. *International Journal of Radiation Biology,* Vol. 69, Issue 3, 1996.

Chapter 15
They Lived To Tell About It

> The A-bomb survivors are living
> longer than the controls despite the
> 400 radiation-induced cancer deaths.
> —Professor John Cameron,
> University of Wisconsin School of Medicine

On the morning of August 6, 1945, Hiroshima, Japan, exploded into the first and largest high-level radiation test laboratory in the world. Three days later, because skies over the Kokura Arsenal on the north coast of Kyushu were overcast, Nagasaki became the second. Most victims died from the intense heat or the blast effect, but hundreds were to succumb later to effects of radiation—while thousands of survivors were instantaneously hit with trillions of neutrons and gamma rays.

In the early 1950s, studies of the effects of radiation were needed by the U.S. military and civilian defense authorities because of the threat of nuclear war with the Soviet Union. A joint U.S.-Japan program was initiated to analyze radiation effects on the populations.

Doses to survivors were estimated by their locations at the time of the blasts, with a "health handbook" being kept by each exposed person in which his medical history was meticulously recorded. Of great importance were the potential mutagenic effects (the original concern over "nuclear monsters"), since it was well known that radiation had a mutational effect on fruit flies and other lower organisms and, therefore, was expected to affect humans at high levels. No such consequences were ever found. In fact, not only were the offspring of survivors *not* negatively affected, but there were benefits that we might now attribute to a hormetic effect of the radiation.

But the primary concern was cancer. Earlier studies of 15,000 people in Great Britain, who had been exposed to upwards of 400 rems in treatment of spinal ailments, had shown a link between high levels of radiation and cancer in a significant percentage of the exposed. The Japanese study, among others, would further refine this relationship to be a 0.018% increase for every absorbed rem. (This is added to the approximately 20% risk of cancer for the average American.) For example a survivor who suffered radiation sickness from an initial pulse of 100 rems would have his or her chance of cancer increased from about 17% to 18.8%. (Remember, this is a dose equal to four times the average lifetime exposure for U.S. residents, ocurring in a few seconds or minutes.)

Indeed, there were several hundred excess cancer deaths in Japan among those who received high doses of radiation.[1] And because of the much greater number of persons receiving lesser amounts (typically equivalent to a lifetime of background radiation absorbed in a few seconds) it was feared, on the basis of the newly adopted Linear No-Threshold and collective dose theories, that these survivors were in for even more tragedy. Leukemia would be kicking in in about three to ten years after exposure, with the other cancers occuring within twenty or, at most, thirty years.

But a funny thing happened on the way to the graveyard: *The bomb survivors were outliving their unexposed peers.* As Dr. Sohei Kondo,[2] put it in his 1993 book entitled *Health Effects of Low-Level Radiation,*[3] "The age-specific rates of death from all causes (observed deaths) [for exposed survivors] in people over sixty years of age were significantly lower than those for people without the health handbook (expected deaths) presumed to be unexposed." In

---

[1] RERF statistics estimate 339 excess cancer deaths (out of 4,687 total cancer deaths) through 1990. John Cameron estimates the projected total at 400.

[2] Mentioned earlier in regard to his *apoptosis* research, Dr. Kondo is professor emeritus of biology, Osaka University and senior researcher, Atomic Energy Research Institute, also in Osaka.

[3] Kinki University Press, Osaka, 1993, and Medical Physics Publishing, Madison, Wisconsin, 1993. Any serious researcher *must* have this book. It is *the* definitive work on the Japanese atomic disaster.

short, the exposed had a significantly lower death rate than those who were fortunately out of town for the war-ending fireworks.

Figure 13 demonstrates the classic hormesis-curve shape for death rates of bomb survivors as a function of absorbed dose. Up to

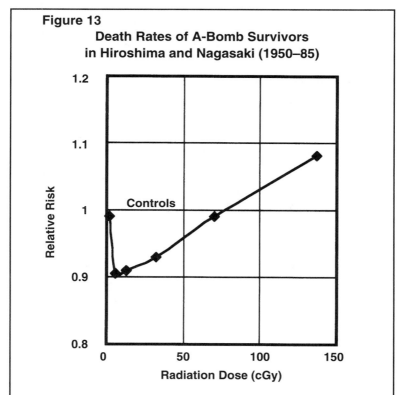

Figure 13
Death Rates of A-Bomb Survivors
in Hiroshima and Nagasaki (1950–85)

Notes:

1. "Relative Risk" is the number of people who have died in a particular exposed cohort compared with (divided by) deaths in a similar group the general population.

2. These data are for male survivors.

3. Only the acute dose resulting from the blast radiation is considered; external and internal doses by fission products, which would enhance the data, are not included.

Source: Mine, M., Okumura, Y., Ichimara, M., Nakamura, T., and Kondo, S. Apparently beneficial effect of low to intermediate doses of A-bomb radiation on human life span. *International Journal of Radiological Biology*, 58:1035, 1990.

approximately 70 rems (or cSv), the death rate for exposed persons is lower than unexposed.[4] (Not shown on this graph, the relative risk for 325 rems is 1.28.) Note that these data were from forty years after Hiroshima and Nagasaki—concluding well past the established latency time for cancer onset from effects of radiation.

In an earlier study, Mine had compared the *observed* deaths of the survivors with the *expected* number and found all age groups from forty-five years to eighty-plus-years had significantly longer life expectancies—just the opposite of what had been predicted by

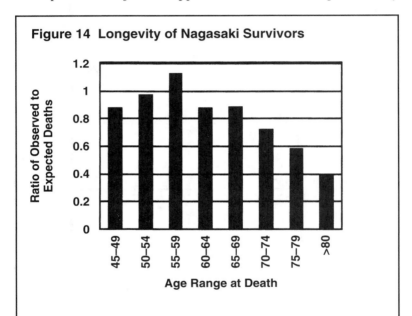

Figure 14 Longevity of Nagasaki Survivors

Note: By definition, the ratio of observed to expected deaths in the general population is 1. In this example, only 38% of the expected number of survivors above eighty years old died, as compared with 100% of a similar group in the general population.

Source: Mine, M., Nakamura, T., Mori, H., Kondo, H., and Okajima, S. The current mortality rates of A-bomb survivors in Nagasaki City. *Japan Journal of Public Health*, 28, p337, 1981. (In Japanese with an English abstract.)

---

[4] Mine et al. Apparently beneficial effect of low to intermediate doses of A-bomb radiation on human life span. *International Journal of Radiological Biology*, 58:1035, 1990.

the LNT. Figure 14 is plotted from "Observed and expected annual rates of deaths (1970–76) from all causes among atomic bomb survivors in Nagasaki." The vertical axis gives the ratio of the observed deaths of male survivors compared with the expected deaths from the general population (who are assumed to be unexposed). Except for the age range of fifty-five to fifty-nine—which had a mortality 12% above the general population—all age groups older than forty-five have less than expected mortality, with the effect increasing with increasing age.[5]

Returning to Kondo,

> The ratio of observed to expected numbers of deaths shows that the mortality of exposed people was slightly lower than or equal to that of unexposed people at all four low to intermediate doses, 1–49, 50–99, 100–149, and 150–199 rad, and that a significant increase in deaths occurred only in the high dose range, 200–599.

This confirms what we already know—that radiation in huge doses is not something to trifle with. But it also suggests that low-level exposure poses no danger and may be helpful.

Leukemia Mortality Among Survivors

Leukemia is a family of cancer involving the white blood cells. With the exception of lymphocytic leukemia—which is often erroneously included—the disease can be induced by ionizing radiation, and hence is the model of a radiation-engendered disorder. One would therefore expect a sizable increase in leukemia as the exposure level increases from the background level of 0.1 cGy as shown in Figure 15. The data—taken from M. Delpha's "Fear of nuclear power could be met with data from Hiroshima"[6] —indicate

---

[5] Data from Mine et al. The current mortality rates of A-bomb survivors in Nagasaki City, *Japan Journal of Public Health,* 28, 337, 1981. N values for data starting at 45–49 are 113, 87, 184, 299, 508, 816, 825, 869.

[6] Delpha, M. *Nuclear Europe,* 42, 3, 1989.

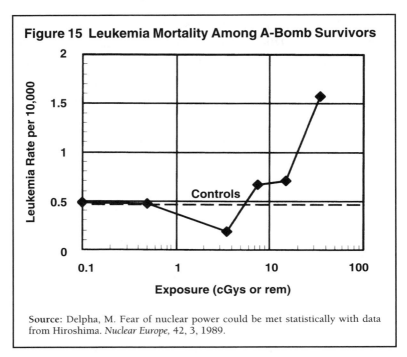

Figure 15 Leukemia Mortality Among A-Bomb Survivors

Source: Delpha, M. Fear of nuclear power could be met statistically with data from Hiroshima. *Nuclear Europe,* 42, 3, 1989.

that the leukemia mortality rate shows a minimum at 3.5 cGy, or about ten times the average annual U.S. background level. Only a single data point gives an indication of hormesis; however, a threshold is positively demonstrated, and a clear difference in the effect of low- and high-level radiation is evident—both in conflict with expectations of the LNT.

All Cancer Mortality in A-Bomb Survivors

The "all cancer mortality" curve of Figure 16, taken from the work of H. Kato, et al.,[7] is noticeably similar to the preceding curve, which depicts leukemia deaths. While the "all cancer" graph (Figure 16) is more indicative of hormesis, both figures are in absolute conflict with the Linear No-Threshold (LNT) theory.

---

[7] Kato H., et al. Dose-response analysis among bomb survivors exposed to low-level radiation. *Health Physics,* 52, 645,1987.

So what has been happening in this continuing saga? By now most Japanese scientists and a sizable portion of the public are aware of the increase in longevity of the bomb survivors. But has this caused any change in the way radiation is viewed by the Japanese regulators? Have we seen any statement from the Radiation Effects Research Foundation (RERF) suggesting a change in the rules that "have been used by numerous international bodies as a basis for establishing radiation protection standards"?[8]

Perhaps I missed the announcements.

It is interesting, however, to observe some of the LNT politics in Japan, as we will see a marked similarity to what is happening in the United States and other countries. As I understand it, the Japanese government is even more bureaucracy-bound than ours. So when we ask the question "Who has an interest in maintaining the present protection standards?" we get the same answer: the

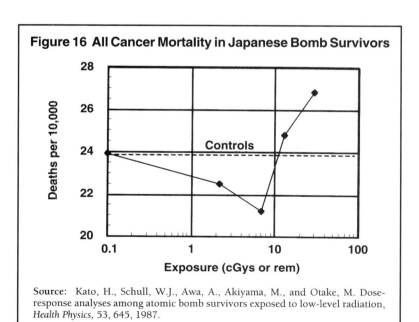

Figure 16 All Cancer Mortality in Japanese Bomb Survivors

Source: Kato, H., Schull, W.J., Awa, A., Akiyama, M., and Otake, M. Dose-response analyses among atomic bomb survivors exposed to low-level radiation, *Health Physics*, 53, 645, 1987.

[8] From "Greetings from the Chairman and Vice-Chairman," RERF web site, www.rerf.or.jp/

government and its minions who are busy, busy, busy at protecting everyone. They couldn't care less about changing the rules to make their "protection" quite unnecessary.

We shouldn't leave Japan without touching on the RERF. Established in 1972 as a continuation of the Atomic Bomb Casualty Commission, the organization has a history of being quite anti-nuclear in its outlook and pronouncements. (Maybe with pictures of total devastation of the two cities on every wall, that is somewhat understandable.) One burr under the saddle of researchers is the secrecy in which exposure data is held even after six decades. Then, too, there are charges that some data have been "adjusted" to give results more like what the 300 or so people with the foundation prefer to see. Funding for the RERF is shared by the Japanese and U.S. governments, the latter being divided between the Department of Energy and the National Academy of Sciences. (One scientist who should know declares that funding has been cut since it became evident that bomb survivors were outliving their unexposed peers, but I have not been able to confirm this.)

While the Japanese government may be reluctant to challenge the LNT, that is not the case for the privately owned utilities and for independent researchers at about a dozen Japanese universities. You will no doubt be amazed and astounded by the current studies from Japan brought to you in chapter 18.

* * * * *

Have you ever wondered about the dangers posed from being a radiation worker in a nuclear power or weapons plant? Maybe *you* should be so lucky! See the next chapter for details.

Chapter 16
Do Nuclear Workers Glow in the Dark?

*Mortality study of plutonium workers at
Rocky Flats involving 7112 workers from
1952 to 1979 gave cancer deaths at 64% of the
expected number in the general population.*
—Nuclear News, December 1981

While the workers building bombs and those involved in electric power generation are in entirely different industries (except in the minds of anti-nuclear protesters), there are many similarities in their work environments. Of particular interest to us are the radiation levels (which are in the area where we would anticipate hormesis), the relatively accurate dosimetry (a fancy scientific word for measuring radiation exposure), and excellent follow-up on the health and longevity of the "participants." We'll look first at two Canadian studies of power plant workers and then at investigations of weapons plant workers by both American and British researchers.

Just in case I forget to mention it three or four times in the next few chapters, *none of these investigations had any intention of even considering the possibility of hormesis.* They were all expecting to prove a positive correlation between radiation and cancer. That's what a "smart" researcher does: makes sure the report comes out to reaffirm what the political authority footing the bill already believes.[1] As you'll see, some researchers *show* data that offer evidence of the hormesis version of dose-response, but they *conclude* that there is a linear relation between radiation and exposure and any particular cancer you'd like to worry about.

---

[1] Most experimentalists are dedicated scientists who let the data speak for themselves. But as in all other facets of life, there are some who play it "smart" to make sure they stay on the government payroll. It is these few that I refer to here.

On to Ontario

In a 1983 study by J.D. Abbatt et al.,[2] the standard mortality ratios (SMRs) of 4,000 nuclear workers were compared with those of 21,000 unexposed "thermal" workers and to those of the general population of nearby Ontario, Canada. Exposures for the nuclear cohort in this investigation, which covered twenty years of plant operation, averaged 7 cGy (7,000 mrad) or about twenty-three years of additional annual background radiation per worker.

Hold the phone. Just what is a "standard mortality ratio" (SMR)? And what does HWE mean? (It hasn't come up yet, but it's getting ready to.) Glad you asked.

First the SMR: If, in the United States, it is observed that 20,000 of the 1 million males aged fifty-nine die per year, we can say that the *rate* of deaths for this group is 2% and that becomes the basis for comparison of other smaller groups of fifty-nine-year-olds. Now let's say we find that in a group of 1,000 fifty-nine-year-old, left-handed Presbyterians, there are only ten deaths, giving us a death rate of 1%. To obtain the *standard mortality ratio* of the Presbyterian lefties we divide its 1% rate by the 2% rate for the total population yielding the ratio 0.50.

If we wanted to know the reason for this lesser mortality ratio, we'd call in an epidemiologist. This special type of statistician might note that most U.S. Presbyterians are Caucasians, who have a lower death rate at age fifty-nine than that of the population in general. Hence race would be considered a *confounding factor* that explains, in part or in total, the difference in the death statistics.

One of the most often used confounding factors in attempts to rebut the hormesis phenomenon is that of the *healthy worker effect* (HWE).

Any employer requiring reliable workers will want to know, at the time of employment negotiations, the health history of the

---

[2] Abbatt, J.D., et al. Epidemiological studies in three corporations covering the Canadian nuclear fuel cycle. From: *Biological Effects of Low Level Radiation,* International Atomic Energy Agency, STI/PUB 646, Vienna, 1983.

prospective employee.[3] Since the healthy applicants, who tend to have a history of less health-related absenteeism, are the first hired, it is logical to assume that the workforce will be healthier than a group of people including those who had applied but were not hired for health reasons. In studies relating to, for instance, tooth decay, we would generally tend to find that the employed contingent had sounder teeth than the total population, some of whom might have lifestyles that didn't include the use of a toothbrush. It would be appropriate in this case to attribute the better dental health to the fact that the individual in question was a "healthy worker."

There is a case, however, where LNT proponents use this confounder to confuse: It is when the employees are *drawn from the same pool* and work in the same or very similar work areas. Since there is no screening test for cancer, there is no way to predict whether the prospective employee will contract it. How, then, can an employee be hired on the basis that he *will not contract cancer later*? We shouldn't discount the HWE, but we shouldn't let others use it to discount the hormesis phenomenon when it is not applicable. Please pardon the interruption, and now back to our story.

The close agreement shown between the thermal worker SMR and that of the general population in Figure 17 would indicate a high degree of reliability for the overall study with a slight degree of "healthy worker effect" (HWE) noted for the non-nuclear cohort. Since there is no HWE in the comparison of nuclear and thermal workers—both being drawn from the same pool—the only difference in the cohorts is the additional radiation exposure of the nuclear workers. This, it would appear, strongly indicates a beneficial effect of low-level radiation exposure—which, of course, is our definition of radiation hormesis.

---

[3] Politicians who pander to certain groups attempt to thwart such reasonable actions—as seen by several Federal laws making health questions illegal.

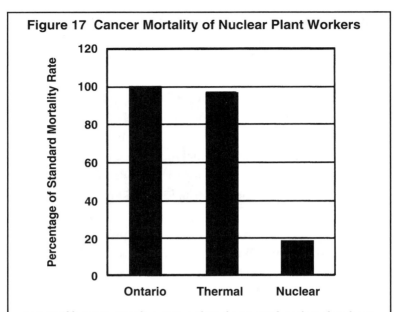

Figure 17 Cancer Mortality of Nuclear Plant Workers

Source: Abbatt, J.D., Hamilton, T.R., and Weeks, J.L. Epidemiological studies in three corporations covering the Canadian nuclear fuel cycle, in *Biological Effects of Low Level Radiation,* International Atomic Energy Agency, Vienna, 351, 1983.

Leukemia in Male Employees of Atomic Energy of Canada, Ltd.

A later study by M.A. Gribbin et al.,[4] examined leukemia mortality of 9,997 male employees of Atomic Energy of Canada, Ltd., with an average exposure of 4.9 cSv (4,900 mrem) compared to 5,504 unexposed co-workers. Figure 18 presents the data in the form of standard mortality ratios for the various types of leukemia.

Commenting on this study, Dr. Jaworowski[5] states:

---

[4] Gribbin, M.A., et al. A study of the mortality of AECL employees, V, the second analysis: Mortality during the period 1950–1985. *Report No. AECL-10615,* Atomic Energy of Canada, Ltd., 1992. Also quoted by Z. Jaworowski in "Stimulating effects of ionizing radiation: New issues for regulatory policy." *Regulatory Toxicology and Pharmacology,* 22:2, 1994.

[5] Zbigniew Jaworowski, professor emeritus at the Central Laboratory for Radiological Protection (Poland) and a member of the U.N. Scientific Committee on the Effects of Atomic Radiation (UNSCEAR).

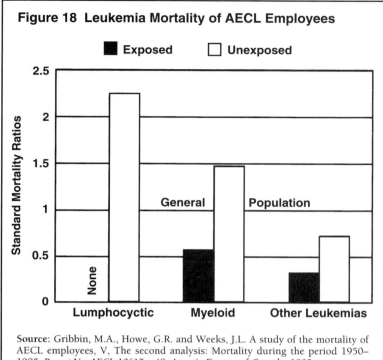

Figure 18 Leukemia Mortality of AECL Employees

Source: Gribbin, M.A., Howe, G.R. and Weeks, J.L. A study of the mortality of AECL employees, V, The second analysis: Mortality during the period 1950–1985, *Report No. AECL-10615*, p48, Atomic Energy of Canada, 1992.

As shown in Table 6 [from which the graph data was taken], the mortality due to all leukemias in the exposed group was only 32% of that in the general Canadian population. The observed mortality among employees of AECL from all cancers and from all non-cancer diseases was also less than expected.

While this is a relatively small study, the consistently lower leukemia mortality rate—previously considered the *established sign of excessive radiation exposure*—seems to be a powerful argument for hormesis at work.

American Weapons Plant Workers

In the first of several planned efforts to combine data on workers at all Department of Energy facilities, this 1989 study was supervised by Dr. Ethel Gilbert of the Pacific Northwest Laboratory.[6] Table III of the report gives a breakdown of Causes of Deaths for 3,368 workers out of a total exposed population of 35,933; these data are summarized in Figure 19. The report summary has some interesting observations:

> These combined analyses provide *no evidence of a correlation between radiation exposure and mortality from all cancer or from leukemia.* Of eleven other specific types of cancer analyzed, multiple myeloma was the only cancer found to exhibit a statistically significant correlation with radiation exposure. Estimates of the excess risk of all cancer and of leukemia, based on the combined data, were negative. [Emphasis added.]

Sounds terrific for LNT opponents! Could it ever be made more clear than by saying "the analyses provide no evidence of a correlation between radiation exposure and mortality from all cancer or from leukemia"? No doubt the report conclusions will cast aspersions on the LNT and set the stage for hormesis research, right? Well, not exactly. It continues:

> *SMRs for all cancers were significantly less than one in all three populations,* probably because of selection bias and other factors related to the healthy worker effect. [Emphasis added.]

You would think that in a study that expects to "provide a direct assessment of health risk" from exposure to low-level radiation, a provision would be made to eliminate the healthy worker effect.

---

[6] Gilbert, E.S., et al. Analyses of Combined Mortality Data on Workers at the Hanford Site, Oak Ridge National Laboratory, and Rocky Flats Nuclear Weapons Plant. *Radiation Research,* 120, 19, 1989.

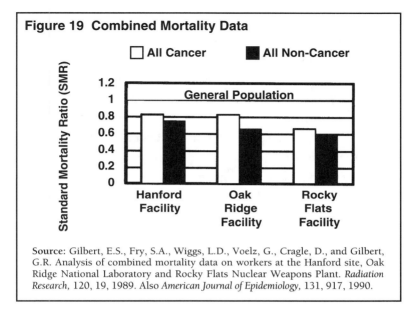

Figure 19 Combined Mortality Data

Source: Gilbert, E.S., Fry, S.A., Wiggs, L.D., Voelz, G., Cragle, D., and Gilbert, G.R. Analysis of combined mortality data on workers at the Hanford site, Oak Ridge National Laboratory and Rocky Flats Nuclear Weapons Plant. *Radiation Research,* 120, 19, 1989. Also *American Journal of Epidemiology,* 131, 917, 1990.

Certainly there were enough non-exposed personnel at these facilities to provide a control cohort. The question is, "Why wasn't this done?"

Ruling out conspiracy and stupidity, one is left with only one possibility I can think of: It was expected that the data would show a cancer mortality rate *higher* than predicted by the standardized rate—which would be the case if the LNT and collective dose were true. No provision was made for the "unexpected result," thus leaving the study with the extremely weak conclusion that the data showed a negative correlation probably because of well, eh, ah… you know. Almost without doubt the researchers were honest, intelligent, dedicated people. But one thing was simply overlooked in analysis of the data: All results that showed evidence of hormesis were simply ignored.

The Most Toxic Substance on Earth?

One of the noisiest guns in the anti-nuclear arsenal has been the cultivated fear of plutonium. "The most toxic substance known to man," so the mantra goes—in complete disregard to toxicity studies showing the element to be about as toxic as caffeine and $1/_{1,000,000,000,000}$ the toxicity of botulism toxin. Even in the health physics field, however, there has been a great deal of concern over inhaled plutonium, because it is an alpha emitter shooting nuclear cannon balls directly into adjacent lung tissue. If you presume radiation is a major cause of cancer, it is only logical to see chronic exposure from an alpha source within the lungs as extremely dangerous. But just as with radon exposure in mining environments, plutonium may not be nearly as dangerous as earlier believed.

During the urgent atomic bomb development period of 1944–45, some workers were exposed to plutonium fumes and extremely fine dust, which accumulated primarily in lung tissue. Twenty-six of these exposed males were followed with regular examinations every five years starting in 1952. When the initial study of these examinations began in 1973,[7] one subject had already died of a heart attack. Anti-nuclear scientists, such as John Gofman, predicted shortened life spans from radiation-induced lung cancer.[8] But apparently, someone forgot to tell the workers.

At the time of the 1986–87 examination period, with an average age of sixty-six years, twenty-two of the twenty-five subjects had refused to die on Gofman's schedule. One had died in an automobile accident, another of a heart attack at age sixty-two, and the third—a pack-a-day-plus smoker—had succumbed to lung cancer in his seventy-second year. (It may be of some interest that this person, identified as Subject #10, was in the lower half of estimated plutonium deposits.)

Because only twenty-six individuals were involved, the study has no statistical significance—which is to say that chance could have been at work selecting certain men who were unusually

[7] Hempelmann, L.H. et al. Manhattan Project plutonium workers. A twenty-seven year follow-up study of selected cases. *Health Physics,* 25, 461, 1973.

[8] Gofman, J.W., *Radiation and Human Health.* Sierra Club Books, San Francisco, 1981.

tolerant to the effects of inhaled plutonium. But the data is also suggestive of a lesser response to plutonium than the LNT dose-response would predict.

Anti-nuclear activists are fond of saying that "a single gamma ray can lead to cancer." Eight of the atomic bomb workers—all living at the end of 1987—had received a dose of more than 2,000,000,000,000,000 alpha particles, which is the equivalent of 8,000,000,000,000,000 gamma rays (assuming a Q of 4). Not only were the "victims" alive, but they were healthier than their peers who weren't lucky enough to inhale plutonium dust more than forty years earlier.

If this study were the only one indicating a biopositive dose-response from plutonium ingestion, it might be written off as an anomoly. But, quoting from a paper by Voelz and Lawrence,[9]

> Other studies of Pu-exposed workers have not demonstrated excesses of lung cancer. In 224 white male Pu-exposed workers, selected on the basis of each having a 1974 estimated Pu deposition in excess of 370Bq (10 nCi), only one death from lung cancer occurred over a 33-year follow-up period. The SMR for lung cancer based on U.S. rates was 0.2 (95% C.I.=0,1.1).

Lest you have forgotten the definition, an SMR of 0.2 means that the lung cancer rate for the workers exposed to plutonium was *one-fifth* that of the general population.

Don't take this as an indication that plutonium is never dangerous when ingested. All the heavy metals are toxic to some degree, and though a relatively benign alpha emitter, it has the potential for being dangerous in large amounts. Several studies noted by Voelz

---

[9] Voelz, G.L. and Lawrence, J.N.P. A forty-two-year medical follow-up of Manhattan Project plutonium workers. *Health Physics*, Vol. 61, 1991. For more information, you might also refer to Voelz, G.L. et al. Mortality study of Los Alamos workers with higher exposures to plutonium. Epidemiology applied to health physics. Proceedings of the Health Physics Society, Albuquerque, N.M. Report CONF-83010, 318, 1983.

in which beagles were exposed to very high doses produced extremely severe consequences. But hormesis is about the *differences in effects of a toxin depending on the dose and/or dose rate.* Evidence in these studies clearly suggests that plutonium may be an effective hormetin.

I Say There, Old Chap

A final study on weapons workers and nuclear power workers comes from England's National Radiological Protection Board. The study, involving 95,100 workers over 3,237,378 person-years was conducted by G.M. Kendall, et al.[10] and caused a recent stir in the United States. T.D. Luckey has taken exception to the manner in which the data was presented, in particular that it dramatically increased the apparent cancer risk by not differentiating between the doses received by certain workers. The English authors have objected to Luckey's objection and are apparently unwilling to undertake any revision[11] that would jeopardize their conclusion. What conclusion is that?

> There is evidence for an association between radiation exposure and mortality from cancer, in particular leukaemia (excluding chronic lymphatic leukaemia) and multiple myeloma, although mortality from these diseases in the study population *was below that in the general population.* [Emphasis added.]

So, considering the data presented in Figure 20, how can the report claim a positive correlation between radiation and cancer? You guessed it: "There is strong evidence of a healthy worker

---

[10] Kendall, G.M., et al. Mortality and occupational exposure to radiation: first analysis of the National Registry for Radiation Workers. *British Medical Journal,* 304, 220, 1992.

[11] Not only are they uninterested in considering a revision, they don't want Luckey doing so either and have refused to supply specific age information, as it might identify particular workers. (Interestingly, in the report, fewer than 2% of the workers requested anonymity.)

effect." Why? Because, according to the report, "Mortality is lower in radiation workers than in the general population of England and Wales—overall and for most specific causes, including cancer."

One might suggest there is a case of circular reasoning here: There is evidence of healthy worker effect since the workers are healthier. As in the study by Dr. Gilbert, no controls of unexposed co-workers were used; nor was any consideration given to the possibility of hormesis.

The LNT dies hard.

For those who have, or may contemplate, working around radioactive materials, you might be pleased to read the following:

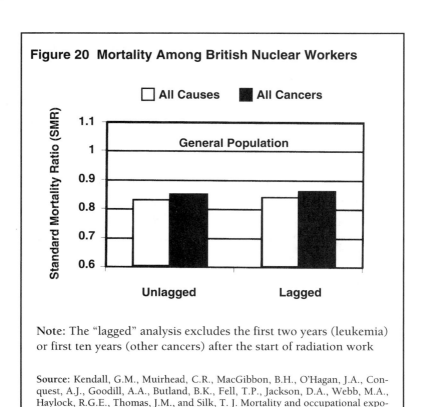

Figure 20 Mortality Among British Nuclear Workers

Note: The "lagged" analysis excludes the first two years (leukemia) or first ten years (other cancers) after the start of radiation work

Source: Kendall, G.M., Muirhead, C.R., MacGibbon, B.H., O'Hagan, J.A., Conquest, A.J., Goodill, A.A., Butland, B.K., Fell, T.P., Jackson, D.A., Webb, M.A., Haylock, R.G.E., Thomas, J.M., and Silk, T. J. Mortality and occupational exposure to radiation: first analysis of the National Registry for Radiation Workers, *British Medical Journal,* 304, 220, 1992.

• There was a 66% decrease in the death rate from infection and parasitic disease in exposed workers at the Savannah River Plant when compared with unexposed controls within the same area.[12]

• Los Alamos workers exposed to greater than 1 mGy (100 mrem) were compared with the U.S. population. The exposed group had only 58% as much total cancer mortality as controls, although brain cancer mortality exceeded controls by 17%. Other cancer categories were: lymphopoietic, 56%; respiratory, 57%; digestive, 67%; leukemia, 75%; no thyroid or bone cancer mortality was found in exposed persons.[13]

• "The total number of deaths experienced by Union Carbide employees in the three Oak Ridge atomic energy facilities over the past 16 years, 1950 through 1965, was compared with the deaths which would be expected or predicted by applying U.S. Bureau of Vital Statistics (BVS) mortality rates to the employee population over this period of time. There were 692 deaths among the plant population over this period, which involved over 200,000 man-years of employment. Based upon the BVS mortality rates, one would have predicted 992 deaths. It is therefore concluded that these employees are experiencing a significantly lower death rate that the average of the white population [the employees were predominately white] throughout the United States."[14]

• "Up-to-date cancer incidence data for those cohorts [weapons plant workers] are reviewed and *continued to show rates below those expected* in the general population. This, in a population of workers exposed during their occupations over many years to radiation doses that would be considered unacceptable today, and

---

[12] Cragle, D.L, et al. Mortality among workers in a nuclear fuel products facility. *American Journal of Industrial Medicine,* 14, 397, 1988.

[13] Acquavella, J.F., et al. A melanoma case-control study at the Los Alamos National Laboratory, *Health Physics,* 45, 587, 1988.

[14] Larson et al. Comparison of Union Carbide employees in Oak Ridge atomic energy facilities with U.S. Bureau of Vital Statistics Mortality, *UCC Report K-A-708,* issued June 9, 1966.

studied as a 'bellwether' for predicting risk to current workers, there is evidence at a cellular level of their having received that exposure, but as yet no evidence of unpredicted harm."[15] [Emphasis added.]

• Mortality studies of plutonium workers at Rocky Flats [Colorado] involving 7,112 workers from 1952 to 1979 gave cancer deaths at 64% of the expected number in the general population.[16]

*   *   *   *   *

I would hate to be a regulator these days and to be required to continually come up with excuses as to why the data are wrong, and why my opinion is right. But then, perhaps things would look differently if my prestige and paycheck were on the line.

---

[15] Berry, R.J., et al. Biological markers, morbidity, and mortality in a long-serving radiation worker population. *American Nuclear Society Transactions,* November 1994.

[16] *Nuclear News,* December 1981, pp. 135–38.

Chapter 17
"Why Don't They Evacuate Norway?" *

 *A question by UN Scientific Committee on the Effects of Atomic Radiation (UNSCEAR) Member Dr. Zbigniew Jaworowski in noting that the limits set for evacuating people from around Chernobyl were below *the average background radiation in Norway,* and far, far below *the high background areas of Norway and many other places in the world.*

ON A PLANET where virtually nothing is distributed equally, we should be surprised if terrestrial sources of background radiation were somehow evenly allocated. And they are definitely not. As noted in Table 10 (in chapter 11), some places have more than 130 times the average background radiation of the United States, and since the U.S. average is considerable higher than the ambient radiation in other locations, there is easily a factor of 150 difference between points on the earth.

Believers in the Linear No-Threshold (LNT) hypothesis tell us that all radiation is dangerous, and that the danger is proportional to the dose received. Hey, since we have all these different levels of background radiation across the globe, all they have to do to prove their theory is to demonstrate that as the background radiation increases, so does cancer incidence—and perhaps even other maladies that we haven't yet even considered might be caused or aggravated by additional exposure.

Sadly (for them), this is demonstrably untrue. More than that. There is a large body of evidence that points in the opposite direction—that we are "underexposed" and that exposure to additional radiation will increase our health and vitality. This chapter intends to show some of that evidence.

China

There are two geographical areas involved in both of the following investigations. The "Low Background" area has a background rate similar to the Gulf Coast states in the United States, i.e., about 100 mrad (0.1 cGy) per year; the "High Background" locations have exposures of approximately 330 mrad—very near the U.S. average. The early study, illustrated in Figure 21, is for relatively large cohorts with a "High" group of 74,000, compared with the "Low" control cohort of 77,000 inhabitants. Since "all radiation is dangerous and unhealthy," we should see the low-background contingent outshining their radiated countrymen in all facets of health and well-being.

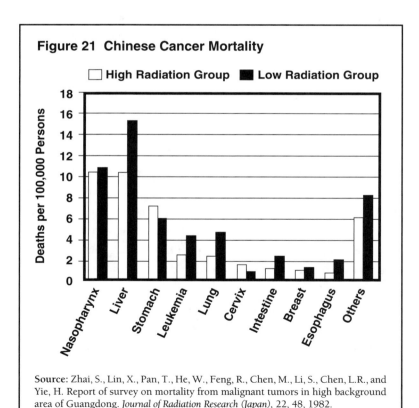

Figure 21 Chinese Cancer Mortality

□ **High Radiation Group** ■ **Low Radiation Group**

Source: Zhai, S., Lin, X., Pan, T., He, W., Feng, R., Chen, M., Li, S., Chen, L.R., and Yie, H. Report of survey on mortality from malignant tumors in high background area of Guangdong. *Journal of Radiation Research (Japan)*, 22, 48, 1982.

Au contraire! The data of Figure 21 support just the reverse. As can be seen in this study by S. Zhai et al.,[1] eight of the ten cancers investigated are higher in the low-radiation group.

A second Chinese study[2] compared several reproduction related criteria for the two groups. In this case the "high" population consisted of 13,425 peasants [their word], with the control "lows" numbering 13,987. Figure 22 shows the relative percentages of reproductive "problems" between the groups. Unless there are some unknown

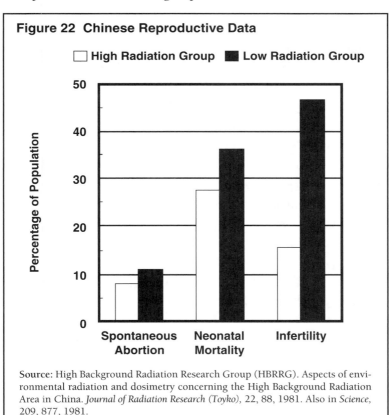

Figure 22 Chinese Reproductive Data

☐ **High Radiation Group** ■ **Low Radiation Group**

Percentage of Population — Spontaneous Abortion / Neonatal Mortality / Infertility

Source: High Background Radiation Research Group (HBRRG). Aspects of environmental radiation and dosimetry concerning the High Background Radiation Area in China. *Journal of Radiation Research (Toyko)*, 22, 88, 1981. Also in *Science*, 209, 877, 1981.

---

[1] Zhai, S., et al. Report of survey on mortality from malignant tumors in high background area of Guangdong. *Journal of Radiation Research (Japan)*, 1982.

[2] HBRRG data in the *Journal of Radiation Research (Tokyo)*, 22, 88, 1981; and also *Science*, 209, 877, 1981.

confounding factors at work here, it is evident that living in a low-background radiation area is not conducive to large families.

If high-background radiation caused an increase in spontaneous abortion, neonatal mortality, or infertility, there would be no end to regulators and the protection bureaucracy attempting to move us all to new locations, dig up the farm, and bury it somewhere. But since all three of these factors are *decreased* with an *increase* in background radiation, no one seems to notice.

India

Indian researchers K.S.V. Nambi and S.D. Soman[3] collected and analyzed cancer mortality data from a number of state hospitals along with the average background radiation in each locality. (Hospitals in Delhi, Kerala, Maharashtra, Pondi, and Tamil Nadu were excluded as they are regional centers that take patients from several states.) A plot of these data, shown in Figure 23, show an unmistakable negative correlation between background radiation and overall cancer mortality. In an extended study,[4] the investigators found a significant inverse relationship (the more radiation, the less cancer) between background radiation and all types of female cancers except those of the mouth and cervix.

Japan

Spring waters have often been found to have significant amounts of dissolved radon. This seems particularly true at springs that are considered "health spas," such as Bad Gastein in Austria, where the activity from radon and its progeny reaches 16,200 pCi/l—a mere 73,600% higher than the "contaminated milk" of such great concern to the media at Three Mile Island. A case in point are the radon

---

[3] Nambi, K.S.V., and Soman, S.D. Environmental radiation and cancer in India. *Health Physics,* 52, 653, 1987.

[4] Nambi, K.S.V., and Soman, S.D. Further observations on environmental radiation and cancer in India. Submitted to *Health Physics,* 1990.

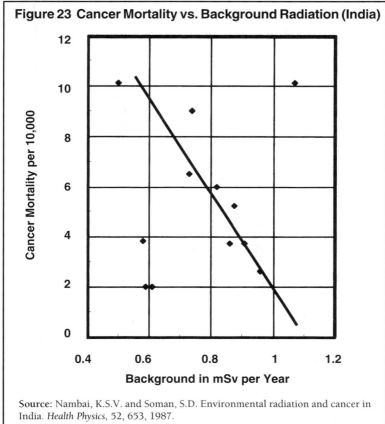

Figure 23 Cancer Mortality vs. Background Radiation (India)

Source: Nambai, K.S.V. and Soman, S.D. Environmental radiation and cancer in India. *Health Physics*, 52, 653, 1987.

springs at Misasa, Japan, where Mifune et al.[5] investigated the prevalence of cancer mortality in Misasa versus that in the nearby town of Beppu Spring, a village with minimal waterborne radon. Also, used as a control, were the Standard Mortality Ratios for all Japan. Data were collected during the period 1952–88.

Stomach cancer mortality is singled out and plotted in Figure 24, since it might be expected from ingesting radon in the water. Obviously there is a significant negative correlation between radon

---

[5] Mifune, M., et al. Cancer mortality survey in a spa area (Misasa, Japan) with a high radon background. *Japan Journal of Cancer Research*, 83, 1, 1992.

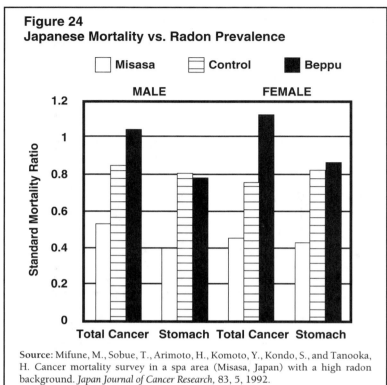

Figure 24
Japanese Mortality vs. Radon Prevalence

Source: Mifune, M., Sobue, T., Arimoto, H., Komoto, Y., Kondo, S., and Tanooka, H. Cancer mortality survey in a spa area (Misasa, Japan) with a high radon background. *Japan Journal of Cancer Research,* 83, 5, 1992.

exposure and cancer—in conflict with the LNT and in good agreement with hormesis expectations.

One unusual feature of the data concerns female responses. Often the observed beneficial effect of radiation is less in females than in males. The Misasa data, however, indicate SMRs for colon/rectum and lung cancer that are significantly lower for women.

Dr. Mifune, regarding a study much like that of Misasa, comments, "Similarly, in one region of Japan with an average indoor level of 35 Bq/m^3, the lung cancer incidence was 51% of that in a low-level radon region (11 Bq/m^3), and the mortality caused by all types of cancers was 37% lower." By the way, to convert Bq/ m^3 to pCi/l, you divide by thirty-seven—which means both of the above

Table 12
Standard Mortality Ratios for Residents of Misasa, Japan

	Male	Female
Total Cancer	.538	.463
Stomach	.400	.452
Colon/rectum	.296	.142
Lung	.475	.187
Leukemia	.445	.534

Source: Mifune, M., et al. Cancer mortality survey in a spa area (Misasa, Japan) with a high radon background. *Japan Journal of Cancer Research*, 83, 1, 1992.

cited areas have relatively low indoor radon. (Just wait until you see what Bernard Cohen says about all this in chapter 20.)

United States

Sources of significant background radiation in the United States are (1) terrestrial sources, such as granite and certain other types of rocks; (2) radon and its progeny from the decay of thorium, uranium, and other radionuclides; and (3) cosmic radiation— which doubles each 6,000 feet in altitude in the temperate latitudes. Several of the Rocky Mountain states, particularly Idaho, Colorado, and New Mexico, have higher than normal levels of each of these categories, combined to make a significant difference between these states and others, especially the Gulf Coast states of Louisiana, Mississippi, and Alabama.

We'll take a look at the cancer rates in these areas (American Cancer Society 1998 data) and compare them with background sources. The Linear No-Threshold (LNT) theory would predict an increase in cancer; the hormesis model forecasts a decrease in cancer—and other diseases or conditions affected by immune competence—as the radiation levels increase in the hormetic range. *You be the judge.*

Jagger investigated[6] the average background exposures and cancer death rates among the 5.84 million people living in Idaho,

---

[6] Jagger, H. Natural background radiation and cancer death in Rocky Mountain states and Gulf Coast states. *Health Physics*, 75(4), 1998.

Colorado, and New Mexico, compared with the same factors for the 10.83 million residents of Louisiana, Mississippi, and Alabama. His results are shown in Figure 25. While the study does not examine the large number of confounding factors that could possibly influence the data, it does illustrate a trend diametrically opposite to the LNT and is strongly indicative of hormesis.

If you are unaccustomed to reading graphical data, please note that Figures 25 and 26 show two different parameters—radiation dose and cancer rate—for two different geographical areas. The scale on the left side of the graph relates to the bar graphs, while the right-hand values pertain to the cancer deaths per 100,000 persons, as shown by the data points and connecting trend line. What is intended to be shown is the *increase* in cancer rate (as evidenced by

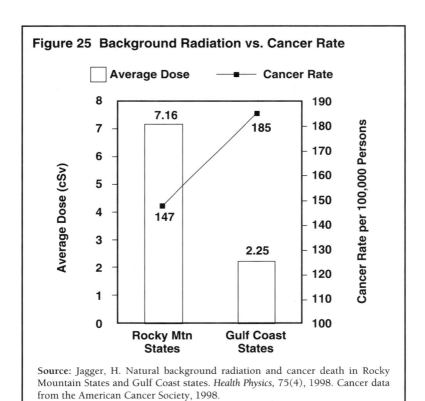

Source: Jagger, H. Natural background radiation and cancer death in Rocky Mountain States and Gulf Coast states. *Health Physics,* 75(4), 1998. Cancer data from the American Cancer Society, 1998.

the upward sloping line) compared with the *decrease* in background radiation indicated by the magnitude of the bar graphs.

A 1994 study by Cohen[7] compares the average radon level and lung cancer rate in the Rocky Mountain states with that in the Gulf Coast states. Radon data come from state agencies, the EPA, and University of Pittsburgh researchers; cancer data are from the American Cancer Society.

Were the data, plotted in Figure 26, to show that lung cancer increased with increasing radon levels, one would have to concede as very likely that the higher residential radon levels were a cause of cancer. Since the evidence shows the exact opposite, one might expect our regulatory agencies to take note and consider revising their policies accordingly. Unfortunately, they apparently don't think they

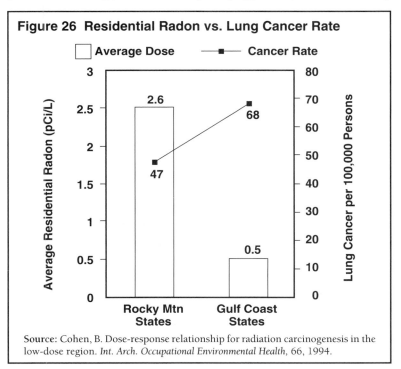

Figure 26 Residential Radon vs. Lung Cancer Rate

Source: Cohen, B. Dose-response relationship for radiation carcinogenesis in the low-dose region. *Int. Arch. Occupational Environmental Health*, 66, 1994.

---

[7] Cohen, B. Dose-response relationship for radiation carcinogenesis in the low-dose region. *Int. Arch. Occupational Environmental Health*, 66, 1994.

should be bothered with such trivial matters as evidence. "It is the radiation protector's task to protect people from radiation, regardless of whether the radiation has bionegative or biopositive effects."

Craig and Seidman[8] studied the rate of leukemia and lymphocytic lymphoma versus altitude in the United States. This, of course, should be a "no-brainer"—everyone *knows* that leukemia is caused by radiation. Since there is about a 4,000 foot difference between the low data points and the high point—and thus a near doubling in cosmic radiation—we will no doubt find, in Figure 27, a doubling of radiation-sensitive cancers like leukemia, right?

Oops. Something is obviously wrong here. I guess it's back to the old drawing board again for the LNTers. Really, this *does* go on and on. Allow me to mention a few of the more interesting cases—without the plots, since I suspect you're starting to tire of the graphs and charts.

Brazil

• No unusual congenital abnormalities, stillbirths, or changes in live births could be found in a Brazilian study of 44,000 pregnancies, even though the background radiation was five to ten times "normal."

• (From the same investigation) "The high terrestrial radiation, 9 mGy/year [900 mrem/yr], in Espirito Santo, Brazil did not affect the fertility of 8,000 couples in this study."[9]

• The beaches of Guarapari have 25%–35% monazite sand giving a dose to vacationers (who bury themselves in it) of 0.03 mGy/hr (at least 30 mrem per ten-hour day—420 mrem for a two-week vacation). Though it's illegal, the tourists steal the rocks and sand for their bedrooms at home.[10]

---

8 Craig, L., and Seidman, H. Leukemia and lymphoma mortality in relation to cosmic radiation. *Blood,* 17, 1961.

9 Freire-Maya, A. and Kreiger, H. Human genetic studies in areas of high natural radiation. *Health Physics,* 34, 61, 1978.

10 Cullen, T.H., et al. Two decades of research in the Brazilian areas of high natural radioactivity. *Radiation Protection: A Systematic Approach to Safety,* Pergamon Press, Oxford, 1980.

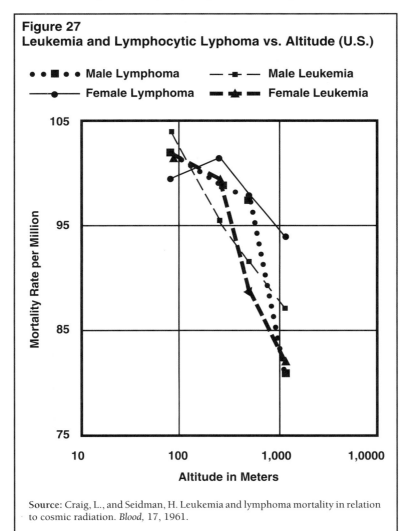

Figure 27
Leukemia and Lymphocytic Lyphoma vs. Altitude (U.S.)

● ● ■ ● ● Male Lymphoma   — ◆ — Male Leukemia
———●——— Female Lymphoma   ■ ▲ ■ Female Leukemia

Source: Craig, L., and Seidman, H. Leukemia and lymphoma mortality in relation to cosmic radiation. *Blood,* 17, 1961.

China

• "In China, a meticulous study measured the radon level for 1 year in the houses of several hundred women with lung cancers and in homes of a similar number of healthy women. The results demonstrated at a 95% confidence level that women who lived in high-level radon houses (more than 350 Bq/m^3) had an 80% lower lung cancer risk than those living in low-level radon houses (4 to 70 Bq/m^3). For perspective, the EPA considers that remedial action at any level down to 70 Bq/m^3 would be cost effective, even for the cost of reducing the level from 150 to 70 Bq/m^3 at about $2 million per hypothetical life saved. (Schiager 1992)."[11]

England

• Mineral collectors have found places near the Cornish town of St. Austell where the background level reaches 4.3 mrem *per minute* (37,700 mrem or 37.7 cGy per year) according to the London-based *Nuclear Issues*. Cornwall and Devon have a cancer incidence well below the British national average.[12]

Finland

• "Conclusions: Our results do not indicate increased risk of lung cancer from indoor radiation exposure."[13]

Germany

• "The observed lung cancer rates of females in high residential radon areas in former uranium mining areas of Southern Saxony are substantially lower than the population average of East Germany. Thus the data from various countries, showing biopositive effects of increased radon levels, can be confirmed in an area which has been closely associated with the history of radiation health effects."[14]

---

[11] Blot, W.J., et al. Indoor radon and lung cancer in China. *Journal of the National Cancer Institute,* 82, 1025, 1990.

[12] Beckmann, Petr. *Access to Energy,* 19, 2, 1991.

[13] Auvinen, A., et al. Indoor radon exposure and risk of lung cancer: a nested case-control study in Finland. *Journal National Cancer Institute,* 88: pp. 966–72, 1996.

[14] Statement by Schuttmann, W. and Becker, K. (of the German Standards Institute), 1998. Reported in *Low Level Radiation Health Effects: Compiling the Data.* Muckerheide, James, ed., Radiation Science and Health, Inc., Needham, Mass., Chapter 1.2.6.3., pp. 1–2.

India

• "While the poorly fed coastal population in Kerala, India, receives 400%–800% more background radiation than neighboring areas, the people have a higher fertility rate with the fewest neonatal deaths of any other Indian state."[15]

United States

• "Studies of populations chronically exposed to low-level radiation, such as those residing in regions of elevated natural radiation, have not shown consistent or conclusive evidence of an associated increase in the risk of cancer."[16] [This statement conflicts with conclusions of the report.]

• In a study of 900,000 U.S. residents with various levels of radium in water supplies, the BEIR was confounded by finding more bone cancer in Chicago—with only 1 mBq/l—than in the areas where the level exceeded 110 mBq/l.[17]

• A multivariant examination of forty-three urban populations of the United States showed a statistically significant negative correlation [more radiation, less cancer] between total cancer mortality and background levels of ionizing radiation.[18]

---

[15] Auxier, J.A., Reactions to BRC. *Health Physics Society Newsletter,* 16, 5, 1988.

[16] From the Executive Summary, Carcinogenic Effects. Biological Effects of Ionizing Radiation Committee [BEIR] of the National Academy of Science, Report V, 1990, p. 5.

[17] From BEIR IV, *Health Risks of Radon and Other Deposited Alpha Emitters,* National Academy Press, Washington, D.C., 1988.

[18] Hickey, R.J., et al. Low level ionizing radiation and human mortality; multi-regional epidemiological studies. *Health Physics,* 40, 625, 1981.

Chapter 18
Take Two Cobalt 60s & Call Me in the Morning

 *If we really believed in the LNT, we would have to conclude that routine use of X-rays for medical purposes would cause 100,000 deaths each year.*
—Richard North, *Alpha,* 1997

R<small>ADIATION AND CANCER</small> are certainly strange bedfellows.

On the one hand there is a great deal of misplaced concern that the almost infinitesimally small emissions from nuclear power plants will cause widespread cancer and induce Farmer Jones's cow to give birth to two-headed calves. Yet when Farmer Jones contracts cancer (no doubt as a result of the power plant), one of the primary treatments is to destroy the cancer cells (which are unusually susceptible to radiation) with X-ray treatments or by implantation of radioactive "seeds" in the cancerous organ. And when Mrs. Farmer Jones has a hyperactive thyroid, she ingests enough iodine 131 to give her body 200 times the radiation dose—in about three weeks—that she receives over her lifetime from the natural background, not to mention the gamma radiation given to her good farmer husband from being next to him in bed. Furthermore, when little Billy Jones is found to have a fatal, inoperative brain tumor, the least invasive treatment is the "gamma knife"—a method of focusing 201 small gamma sources, which, individually, are too weak to cause any harm to anyone but the most fervent anti-nuke. Yet when they are concentrated on the offending growth together they have the power to vaporize it…and Billy goes home that afternoon completely cured. Is that a miracle or what?

However, we are not going to discuss this type of radiation therapy, since it involves the transfer of considerable amounts of energy to tissues—particularly tumors or cancers—in an attempt to destroy them or reduce their functionality. Instead, we will be concerned about the effects of comparatively tiny amounts of radiation whose purpose is to provoke the immune system into stepping up its action on the cellular level.

You may note in this chapter that virtually all of the current experimental activity mentioned is occurring in Japan, where the work of Dr. Luckey is revered—since, I suspect, it explains so much of what is happening to bomb survivors. But the Japanese have taken the matter much further, including hormetic augmentation of high-level therapies and measurement of the physiological reactions to radiation—including one that gives credence to an unusual treatment for arthritis that dates back to Roman times.

Keeping Abreast of the Evidence

Breast cancer is a pretty depressing matter. An estimated 44,300 women (and several thousand men) will die of breast cancer this year. It is second only to lung cancer as a cause of cancer death among women. Increased use of mammography is one of the reasons for the decline in death rates. In 1992 (the most recent statistics I could find), 67% of women over forty reported having at least one screening—up from only 22% in 1979.

But sadly, many women are still hesitant to have *regular* mammography examinations, often because they fear that X-rays from the mammograms will increase their chances for cancer. Doing their own *risk assessment,* they conclude the risk from "late detection" is less than that from radiation. And who is to blame them, in light of the commonly accepted dictum that all radiation is dangerous and cumulatively so? Besides, it costs time and money to have a mammogram—at least worrying about cancer is cheap.

"So," you say, "they should just consult a professional and ask about the dose they will receive from the mammogram and make the decision on that basis." Not as simple as that may sound. In researching this chapter I called four local mammography clinics with what I thought was a pretty simple question: "What is the dose of radiation received by a woman in the process of having a mammogram?" I had seen a figure before, but it seemed high to me.

I spoke with two mammography technicians and one nurse who relayed messages from their radiologists. The unanimous answer: "We don't know." One of them, however, was kind enough to put me in touch with a local health physicist, who said the dose was "negligible"—but, even better, offered to lend me some of his reference books. In one, I was able to find the range of exposures to a "gland" (their quotation marks) at a depth of 3 cm to be 0.04 to 0.49 cGy (40 to 490 mrem), which was consistent with the 0.15 cGy figure I had found earlier and was trying to confirm.

But the information I had was perplexing, as it mentioned the dose as 150 mrem *per breast.* It was much like the confusion I had when learning that radon gave an exposure of 24,000 mrem/year to the bronchial epithelium (which, of course, you now know is the windpipe). The borrowed volumes were quite illuminating. I found there is an official **weighting factor** that, when multiplied by the *local* dose gives the **effective dose equivalent.** And what does this tell you? It tells you the increase in your chances of contracting cancer *if the Linear No-Threshold theory were true!*

Using a weighting factor of 0.15 for each breast,[1] a 150 mrem per breast exposure would be an equivalent "whole body" exposure totaling 45 mrem (0.045 cSv.) The figure—in my opinion—means nothing, but if we pretend it is accurate we can use it as a starting point for a "conventional" analysis.

Published in the *New England Journal of Medicine* in 1989,[2] an investigation by A.B. Miller and associates charted the doses received by 31,710 women who were irradiated in the course of repeated fluoroscopic examinations between 1930 and 1952. In

---

[1] Exposure of the U.S. Population from Diagnostic Medical Radiation, NCRP Report #100, National Council on Radiation Protection and Measurements, Bethesda, Md.

[2] Miller, A.B., et al. Mortality from breast cancer after irradiation during fluoroscopic examination in patients being treated for tuberculosis. *New England Journal of Medicine,* 321, 1285, 1989.

Figure 28

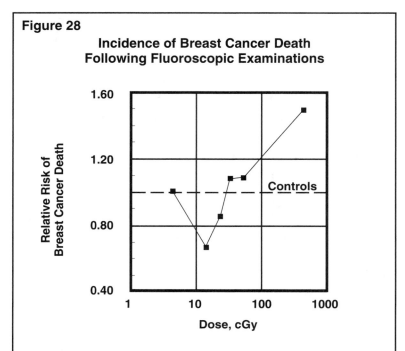

**Incidence of Breast Cancer Death
Following Fluoroscopic Examinations**

Source: Miller, A.B., Howe, G.R., Sherman, G.J., Lindsay, J.P., Yaffe, M.J., Dinner, P.J., Risch, H.A., and Preston, D.L. Mortality from breast cancer after irradiation during fluoroscopic examination in parients being treated for tuberculosis. *New England Journal of Medicine,* 321:1285, 1989.

this Canadian study, one group—in Nova Scotia—was fluoroscoped facing the X-ray source. This results in a dose to the breast approximately twenty-five times that when faced away. The women facing the source had a significant increase in cancer risk—it tripled for each 100 cGy (100,000 mrad) of radiation absorbed.

The balance of the study was for all other provinces, with the results presented in Figure 28. Before going on, please remember that a normal annual U.S. background dose is 0.3 cGy. with the first data point on the graph at 5 cGy—about thirteen times this amount. The *minimum mortality* rate is at a value fifty times the annual background dose or the equivalent (using *their* figures) of 100 mammography exams.

On the basis of this evidence—which is almost certainly conservative, since the dose *rate* for fluoroscopy is much higher and, therefore, considered more traumatic to the breasts than present mammography techniques—women should have four or five mammograms per year.

Does that sound strange? That's *nothing* compared with the most unusual aspect of the study, namely its conclusion: The authors completely ignored the most statistically significant data points in the entire investigation, namely the 34% reduction in relative risk at 15 cGy and the 15% reduction at 25 cGy. Myron Pollycove, M.D.,[3] remarked regarding this omission,

> The decreased RR [risk rate] of breast cancer produced by low dose, low level radiation were rejected *a priori* by the choice of mathematical models that extrapolate the dose-risk relation from high dose exposures to low dose exposures.

To most of us that simply means the researchers, for whatever reason, chose to "spike" all results that indicated hormesis. Why? Probably because they were not even *considering* bio-positive data; they were looking for harmful effects...period. Pollycove continues,

> Nine hundred excess deaths from breast cancer are predicted theoretically from the exposure of one million women to 0.15 Gy. However, the quantified low dose data predicts with better than 99% confidence limits that instead of causing 900 deaths, a dose of 0.15 Gy would prevent 10,000 deaths in these million women.

---

[3] We met Dr. Pollycove back in chapter 2. But since he is such an important player in the LNT controversy, allow me to remind you that he is professor emeritus in Laboratory Medicine and Radiology at the University of California at San Francisco, head of Nuclear Medicine at San Francisco General Hospital, as well as a visiting medical fellow on the Nuclear Regulatory Commission.

Pardon me, but do you understand what this man—who has possibly the most impressive credentials in this entire debate—is saying? He is proclaiming that there is unmistakable evidence of hormesis in this study, which, if acted upon, might be developed into an effective weapon against breast cancer in *millions of women, thousands of whom will die needlessly because of a theory that was never intended to apply to low-level radiation!* It is a pity, a shame, a disgrace that the current ingrained reliance by regulators on the Linear No-Threshold hypothesis makes even a consideration of studying the hormesis phenomenon extremely difficult, if not impossible.

That Temperamental Thyroid Gland

Most of our organs—like our hearts and kidneys—either work or they don't. Our thyroid gland, however, either can refuse to work hard enough (hypothyroidism), or can put out too many hormones (hyperthyroidism)—either of which can make life miserable. Those who are the victims of excessive thyroxin have several choices to reduce production of this hormone: whacking away at the thyroid with a scalpel, drugging it into submission, or introducing radioactive iodine 131 into the body, which rushes directly to the gland and essentially wounds it, thus decreasing its activity.[4]

A study by B.M. Dobyns, et al.[5] observed the prevalence of thyroid cancer incidence in 35,000 hyperthyroid patients out to twenty years after treatment. Some 1,200 of these were treated with drugs, with another 12,000 having undergone surgical treatment. The majority, about 22,000, were subjected to very high doses of

---

[4] Iodine 131 is also used both for diagnosis of thyroid function and, in the case of a malignancy, "ablating" or "burning up" the organ. The latter procedure has made thyroid cancer probably the most successfully treatable of all malignancies.

[5] Dobyns, B.M., et al. Malignant and benign neoplasms of the thyroid in patients treated for hyperthyroidism: a report of the cooperative thyrotoxicosis therapy follow-up study. *Journal of Clinical Endocrinological Metabolism,* 1974.

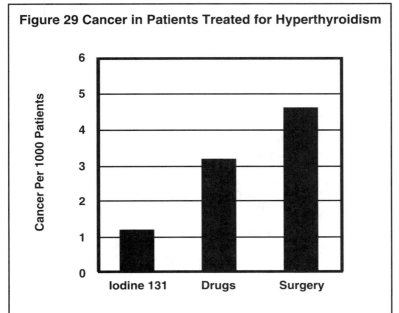

Figure 29 Cancer in Patients Treated for Hyperthyroidism

Source: Dobyns, B.M., Sheline, G.E., Workman, J.B., Tompkins, E.A., McConahey, W.M., and Becker, D.V. Malignant and benign neoplasms of the thyroid in patients treated for hyperthyroidism: A report of the cooperative thyrotoxicosis therapy follow-up study. *Journal of Clinical Endocrinological Metabolism,* 38:976, 1974.

[131]I—on the order of 50,000 mrem or 50 cSv. One would logically expect rampant cancer in these individuals on the basis of the LNT. But it's (another) miracle! As Figure 29 indicates, not only did radiation *not* result in a high malignancy rate, but it seems to have had a hormetic aftermath. Gee, perhaps this can be explained by the "healthy patient effect."

It's Not Too Late to Radiate!

We are all aware of the use of high-energy radiation to kill cancer cells within the body. The problem has always been in not wiping out more of numerous good ones while attempting to eliminate the radiation-susceptible cancer cells. After years of ex-

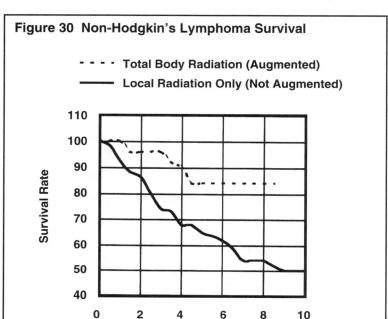

Figure 30 Non-Hodgkin's Lymphoma Survival

- - - - **Total Body Radiation (Augmented)**
────── **Local Radiation Only (Not Augmented)**

Source: Sakamoto, Kiyohiko. Survival of stage I and II of non-Hodgkin's lymphoma treated local irradiation only or combined treatment of TBI* and local irradiation. *Journal of JASTRO,* Sept. 1997.

An earlier report on the same subject with wider availability is: Sakamoto, K and Myojin, M. Fundamental and clinical studies on tumor control by total body irradiation. *American Nuclear Society Transactions,* 75, 404, 1996.

*Total Body Irradiation.

periments with mice, Dr. Kiyohiko Sakamoto[6] is giving hormesis-level doses along with his X-ray treatment for non-Hodgkin's lymphoma.[7] Figure 30 shows the latest update of his work.

Patients with augmentation doses—typically 10 rad (10 cGy) by X-ray three times a week for five weeks—had a survival rate 68%

---

[6] A physician and professor emeritus at Tohoku University.

[7] Sakamoto, K. and Myojin, M. Fundamental and clinical studies on tumor control by total body irradiation. *American Nuclear Society Transactions,* 75, 404, 1996.

greater than the patients without augmentation. It seems odd to me that the hormetic level radiation is given after, not prior to the larger suppressive dose. But then, it's hard to argue with success.

We're Out of Copper, But How About a Zirconium Bracelet?

Among the cruelest deceptions perpetrated upon people by other people are those having to do with phony medical aids, sham healing potions, "miracle" cures, and other forms of snake oil. It just seems to be my nature to suspect the worst when even the most trustworthy appearing people suggest to me some "cure" that has somehow been overlooked by pharmaceutical manufacturers who spend a few billion dollars a year on research—but is well known to granny and the girls working down in the lingerie department. This isn't to say that it doesn't happen, but these "cures" are certainly suspect from the start with me. And so it was when I first heard about the "Free Enterprise Mine" and its claim to have a beneficial effect on arthritis, bursitis, and a dozen or so other debilitating conditions.

For starters, I didn't like the name. Not because I don't like the free-enterprise system, but because I do. It seemed to me that charlatans might be using a good name to disguise another of those despicable medical deceptions. This was early in my attempt at writing this book—and I didn't think any more about it for several months. By then I knew about the high radon content of many European spas and those at Bad Gastein in particular. To me, these resorts, which compete for having the highest radiation level, just showed that our fears of radon and low-level radiation were what I had already suspected: contrived and ridiculous.

What I didn't know was that the major "cures" offered by such health resorts as the "Thermal Galleries" (a former gold mine and only one of the many spas in the Bad Gastein area) were for "rheumatic, arthritic, and scoliotic disease." What was described in their advertisements was much like what I had heard about the Free Enterprise Mine, with one big difference: The spas had a two-thousand year history of arthritics coming there for relief. Still, the placebo effect and mass hypnosis didn't start with the twentieth century. I don't enjoy being fooled, and what's more, I didn't plan to be a shill for anyone bent on fooling others. Skepticism reigned.

Only very recently did I learn of the Japanese research on the hormonal reactions to inhalation of radon. (The test animals in these experiments were rabbits rather than mice.) As shown in Figure 31, there were marked increases in both beta-endorphins and m-enkephalins in the test animals. Those who know about such things claim that the former is a pain reliever, while the latter hormone creates a feeling of well-being.

It dawned on me that I now had evidence from three continents leading to the same conclusion: that radon inhalation has a positive effect on arthritic diseases.

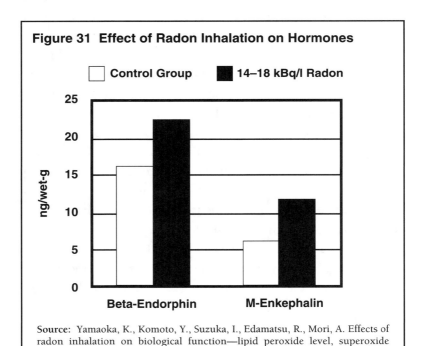

Figure 31 Effect of Radon Inhalation on Hormones

Source: Yamaoka, K., Komoto, Y., Suzuka, I., Edamatsu, R., Mori, A. Effects of radon inhalation on biological function—lipid peroxide level, superoxide dismutase activity, and membrane fluidity. *Arch Biochem Biophys.* 1993 Apr; 302(1):37-41.

I remembered that someone had sent me a book on the Free Enterprise Mine, which I had carefully filed in the "probably won't need this" box. The name of the book was *Arthritis and Radioactivity*,[8] by Wade V. Lewis, the original owner of the mine. I learned that it didn't start out as any kind of treatment facility, but as a uranium mine in 1949. By chance, the wife of a visiting engineer went down in the mine with him and found to her amazement that her debilitating arthritic condition had improved. She convinced a friend in similar circumstances to return with her to see if this was "for real." Apparently it was, as the mine has flourished ever since.

The best thing about the book is its tone. It is not written in a "This is the way it is" and "This is what's happening" manner. It's more like "This is the way it appears" and "Perhaps this is the cause." The author, who died in 1974, was not a scientist but had learned a great deal about radiation and was trying to put the pieces together. If only he had had Luckey and Pollycove around at the time, it's no telling what the trio could have accomplished.

On August 27, 1999, there were a number of scientists on the way to a "Nuclear Technology—Bridging the Millennia" conference in Jackson, Wyoming. Among the speakers was Sadao Hattori, a Ph.D. in nuclear engineering who is vice-president and director of nuclear energy research at the Central Research Institute of the Electric Power Industry (CRIEPI) of Japan. Earlier, while compiling quotations from a large number of scientists (by which I hoped to show the depth of scientific criticism of the LNT and support for hormesis research), I ran across this 1996 quotation from the animated and dedicated "hormesian,"[9] Dr. Hattori.

We [CRIEPI] are now carrying out experimental activities on the effects of low-dose radiation on mammals. After several years of

---

[8] Available from Free Enterprise Mine, P.O. Box 67, Boulder, MT 59632. Email: hlthmine@mt.net.

[9] Your author's first (and probably last) attempt at coining a word.

research activities, we are recognizing Luckey's claim. Some basic surveys, including Hiroshima-Nagasaki survivors and animal experiments in Japan, have brought us exciting information on the health effects of low-dose radiation.

He went on to say that results for their research would be forthcoming. Let me tell you: Dr. Hattori delivers. In his paper delivered at the 1999 Boston conference of the American Nuclear Society, the nuclear scientist spoke on the following areas being explored by Japanese researchers:

- Okumura's longevity of survivors exposed to low dose A-bomb radiation
- Sakamoto's non-Hodgkin's lymphoma successes
- Onishi's reports of enhancing the p53 tumor suppression gene
- An update on Mifune's Misasa Radon Spring study
- Yonezawa's research on Adaptive Response Windows
- Miyachi's work on stress moderation and pain relief
- Yamaoka's studies of hormonal and adrenaline increases

There is one more study by Yamaoka with which an enterprising tabloid reporter could write his own ticket—if he could only understand a little science.

Yamaoka has found that radiation has a beneficial effect on cell membrane permeability, which in turn has a positive effect on the life of a particular cell. Stimulatory radiation equals high permeability, no wrinkles, no aging—and before this, relief from arthritis and related conditions. Rather interesting stories, wouldn't you say? Gee, I wonder where the reporters have gone.

* * * * *

Allow me to give you just a few snippets on other subjects related to both medicine and radiation:

- "Court-Brown and Doll (1958) using a standard cohort technique, analyzed the mortality of radiologists belonging to the 2 major radiological societies in the United Kingdom through 1956.

Radiologists joining radiological societies after 1920 would have had 176 deaths if they had the same life expectancy as the general population, or 169 deaths if their life expectancy was the same as that of physicians in general. Only 145 deaths were recorded."[10]

• A study of 100,000 female radiology technicians, with a mean follow-up time of twenty-nine years since certification, showed no association for breast cancer with vocational experience in radiotherapy, nuclear medicine, or fluoroscopy.[11]

• "A critical review of the literature leads to the conclusion that at the radiation doses generally of concern in radiation protection,[12] protracted exposures to low linear energy transfer (LET) radiation does not appear to cause lung cancer. *There is, in fact, indication of reduction of the natural incidence.*"[13] [Emphasis added.]

Finally, there is the connection between cancer and the application of radium to watch dials, which is fairly notorious in medical texts. The women (there were only about a dozen men in this vocation) touched their tongues to their brushes while painting, thereby receiving a large internal dose. Just as in the case of H-bomb test fallout victims, I thought all the painters died early deaths from radiation-induced cancer. Perhaps the literature left you with the same erroneous impression.

• "The absence of leukemia and other potential radiogenic cancers in the population of highly exposed radium dial painters—from both internal and external radiation—contradicts the LNT; moreover, *the increased longevity of these workers* has been noted, but

---

[10] Henry, Hugh (Oak Ridge National Laboratory). Is all radiation harmful? *Journal of the American Medical Association,* 16, 671, 1961.

[11] Boice, J.D., et al. U.S. National Cancer Institute risk of breast cancer evaluation. *Journal of the American Medical Association,* Vol. 274, No. 5, 1995.

[12] Greater than 2 gray (or 200,000 mrad).

[13] Rossi, H. and Zaider, M. Radiogenic lung cancer: the effects of low doses of low linear energy transfer (LET) radiation. *Radiation Environmental Biophysics,* 36, 1997.

competent documentation does not exist at this time."[14] [Note: Support for study of these workers has been cancelled.]

*   *   *   *   *

Before turning the page, consider for a moment what evidence it would take to make you a "hormesian." (Not to worry, I promise not to use that word again.)

---

[14] Kondo, Sohei. (Senior Researcher, Atomic Energy Research Institute, Osaka) *Health Effects of Low-Level Radiation.* Kinki University Press, Osaka, and Medical Physics Publishing, Madison, Wisc., 1993.

Chapter 19
Something's Fishy in the Shipyard

*The nuclear worker groups had
a lower death rate from all causes, leukemia,
and LHC than the non-nuclear workers.*
—Professor Emeritus Myron Pollycove, M.D.,
University of California at San Francisco,
Medicine and Radiology

Suppose you're not convinced about the concept of radiation hormesis and want to do a statistical analysis to settle the matter in your own mind. What is your concept of a "convincing" study? How would you design an experiment so that you would have no doubt about the trustworthiness of the results? Some safeguards I'd like to see would be:

1. The study would have to be supported by deep pockets, because there would be a lot of expense in collecting and analyzing the mountains of data involved.

2. I would want those in charge of the actual research (as opposed to those who are paying for it) to be scientists from a reputable institution.

3. There must be a very large number of exposed persons and the same order of unexposed controls, with both chosen randomly from the same employment pool in order to make the study statistically meaningful and to avoid any possible "healthy worker effect."

4. The doses to the individuals would have to be as accurately known as possible, at least up to industrial or military standards.

5. The study would have to look at not only cancer but also total mortality, in order to test the hypothesis that radiation hormesis not only might reduce cancer, but also might

lessen the effects of infectious diseases and other immune system breakdowns.

6. Finally, I would want the researchers to believe that they were attempting to measure a positive correlation between radiation and disease, without even suspecting that any hormesis effect was of interest.

The following investigation at Johns Hopkins meets all my criteria.

Some Background for the Study

A 1978 report[1] raised the question of low-dose ionizing radiation risk to nuclear workers at the Portsmouth, New Hampshire, shipyard. In 1980, a U.S. Department of Energy contract was granted to the Department of Epidemiology at The Johns Hopkins University to study "Health Effects of Low-Level Radiation in Shipyard Workers."[2] It is apparent from the introduction that this was expected to be a confirmation of the earlier "limited study" and certainly had nothing to do with verification of the hormesis principle—which it ended up being.[3]

The study involved an initial pool of 700,000 workers—including 108,000 nuclear workers—at two private and six government shipyards. Most were weeded out because of missing or incomplete records. Then too, many of the non-nuclear workers did not work in a shipyard during the time when nuclear overhauls were done and were therefore not considered to be comparable to nuclear workers. Two other steps—a crosscheck of records and a question-

---

[1] Identified as "Najarian, 1978" in the Johns Hopkins Report Introduction, referring to brief study done by Dr. Thomas Najarian, a hematologist at the Boston Veterans Administration hospital.

[2] DOE Contract Number DE-AC02-79EV10095.

[3] The term "radiation hormesis" had not even been used yet, as Luckey's first book was still a year or two away when the contract was awarded.

naire to the worker or next of kin—pared the list down to 72,356 qualified subjects. Workers were divided into three categories:

• Those with duties *not* involving radiation, the Non-Nuclear Workers (NNW's—or in our case, the **Nones**). This group of 33,352 workers was used as the control.

• Those who had cumulative exposure of less than 500 mrem. These were termed NW<0.5, which we will call the **Lows**, and totaled 10,462 workers.

• Those with cumulative exposures greater than or equal to 500 mrem. They were referred to as NW>0.5, which we'll refer to as the **Highs**, numbering 28,542 workers.

Results of the study were tabulated to show mortality ratios of the above cohorts from various types of cancer and from all causes. By the way, although the Johns Hopkins report to the Department of Energy was completed nearly fifteen years ago, the Energy Department has yet to acknowledge the results and issue its report on the study.

And Now the Envelope, Please...

When the data were analyzed and tabulated, there must have been a number of stunned Johns Hopkins Ph.D.s wondering what had happened. They started out to show the adverse effects of gamma radiation and ended up showing that it enhanced healthfulness.

The first page of the "Summary of Findings" tells the story:

> The all cause mortality is highest for the NNW [Nones] group and lowest for the NW>0.5 [Highs] which certainly does not suggest that radiation causes a general risk of health. In fact, in the NW>0.5 group, the mortality is only 76 percent of that of the general population and is significantly lower than would be expected.

Following these statements are eight pages of possible explanations of what may have happened to give such unexpected results. One suggestion was to use the Lows as the comparison group instead of the Nones, but even this still has the higher exposed group with the lowest overall death rate…not what was expected. An attempt to explain away the unusual with the usual "healthy worker effect" was mentioned, though without much enthusiasm. But nothing in the report even got close to explaining the numbers printed in the report under "Actual Data."

Remedial Acronyms

There are a couple abbreviations used in Table 13 and/or Figure 32 that may need reminders. **SMR** stands for **standardized mortality ratio** and compares the death rate of a group in question with that of an age-adjusted population of peers. In this study, for

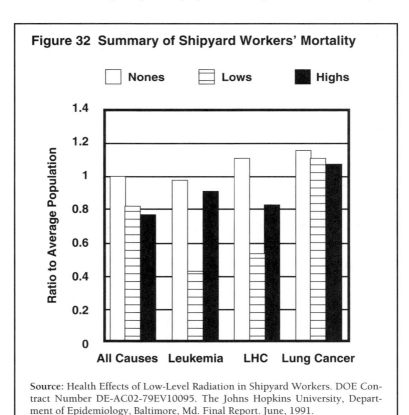

Figure 32 Summary of Shipyard Workers' Mortality

Source: Health Effects of Low-Level Radiation in Shipyard Workers. DOE Contract Number DE-AC02-79EV10095. The Johns Hopkins University, Department of Epidemiology, Baltimore, Md. Final Report. June, 1991.

instance, it is seen that the Nones group has a SMR of 1.00. This means it exactly corresponds with the general population data accumulated over many years by the U.S. Bureau of Vital Statistics—just what you might expect from so large a population sample.

Table 13

Summary of Mortality, Standard Mortality Ratio (SMR), and 95% Confidence Interval* for Shipyard Workers

CAUSE OF DEATH:	NW>5 "Highs"	NW<5 "Lows"	NNW "Nones"
All Causes	2,797	1,168	4,453
SMR	0.76	0.81	1.00
95% Confidence*	0.73, 0.79	0.76, 0.86	0.97, 1.03
Leukemia	21	4	29
SMR	0.91	0.42	0.97
95% Confidence*	0.56, 01.39	0.11, 1.07	0.65, 1.39
LHC	50	13	29
SMR	0.82	0.53	1.10
95% Confidence*	0.61, 1.08	0.28, 0.91	0.88, 1.37
Mesothelioma	18	8	10
SMR	5.49	6.14	2.54
95% Confidence*	3.03, 8.08	2.48, 11.33	1.16, 4.43
Lung Cancer	237	98	306
SMR	1.07	1.11	1.15
95% Confidence*	0.94, 1.21	0.90, 1.35	1.02, 1.29

Source: Johns Hopkins Final Report, Health Effects of Low-Level Radiation in Shipyard Workers, June 1991, Table 4.1, p 344.

* The use of 95% confidence limits is a method to show the range of statistically possible values on either side of the most probable value.

You should remember that the SMR has nothing to do with the number of deaths from a particular risk—just the ratio of deaths in, say, nuclear-plant workers to (divided by) the number of deaths expected in individuals of similar ages and backgrounds.

LHC stands for Lymphatic and Hematopoietic Cancer, which relates to cancers of the lymph nodes and the formation of blood in the body.

A fifth cancer category was not plotted with the rest of the data in Figure 32: the SMR for mesothelioma. Table 13 indicates that both exposed groups showed more than twice the mortality of the unexposed workers. The report suggests, however, that this high ratio was due to both a low (and therefore statistically inaccurate) number of deaths from this cause, and the exposure of both radiation worker groups to environments laden with *amphibole* fibers— the imported, dangerous form of asbestos. (Not to be confused with the benign *chrysotile* variety.)

Don't Let Data Get in the Way of a "Made Up" Mind

What is the significance of this report? Professor Emeritus John Cameron of the University of Wisconsin Medical School puts it in perspective:

> This study is probably the best scientific evidence, of many scientific data sources, to show that low levels of ionizing radiation are without health hazard. The results clearly contradict the conclusions of BEIR[4] that even small amounts of radiation have risk (in BEIR V and earlier reports), which have been largely based on the data from the Japanese atomic bomb survivors, who largely received their radiation exposures in very brief, high dose rate conditions and who are also now demonstrating that effective radiation health effects thresholds exist in the range of 20 to 200 rem [20 to 200 cGy].

---

[4] American Academy of Science Biological Effects of Ionizing Radiation committee.

It is commonplace for us to read various national polls in the newspapers based on 1,044 or so interviews. Presidents and tax-peasants alike make decisions from the opinions of a group of individuals that wouldn't fill one side of a high school basketball gymnasium. Yet in the United States, with a sample size of about 1,000, the statistical error is on the order of 5%. Compare that sample size with the *72,000 individuals* evaluated in the in-depth scientific survey being presented here. Yet the Department of Energy hasn't bothered to explain why their own study flies in the face of their regulatory policy.

* * * * *

Permit me to elaborate on just a few points. Certainly you are welcome to draw your own conclusions from the surprising (to the researchers, anyway) Johns Hopkins data, but here are the top three things that jump out at me in response to this data:

• Why would 28,000 workers, with the same backgrounds as the guys they stood with in the hiring line, have 24% fewer deaths than their non-nuclear buddies?

• Except for mesothelioma, which was attributed to other causes, the *exposed* individuals invariably had a lower mortality than *unexposed.* This is precisely the opposite of what the LNT hypothesis would predict.

• While the lung cancer rate of all workers was higher than that of the general population—presumably since more industrial workers smoke cigarettes than do coaches and preachers—it is very interesting that these data parallel others that show that the exposure of lung tissue to radiation reduces lung cancer. The alpha radiation from radon and plutonium, in particular, seems to do a good job. (No, I'm really *not* kidding.)

* * * * *

Get ready for a treat. You are about to meet Bernie Cohen.

Chapter 20
Before You Spend $4,000 to Shorten Your Life

The observed lung cancer rates of females
in high residential radon areas in
the former uranium mining areas of
Southern Saxony are substantially lower than
the population average of East Germany.
—Professor Klaus Becker,
German Standards Institute

Bᴇʀɴᴀʀᴅ Cᴏʜᴇɴ, ᴅᴏᴄᴛᴏʀ of science and professor emeritus at Pittsburgh University, is a liberal Democrat.[1] I probably would disagree with everything he believes in politically. But Dr. Cohen is also a scientist. He is convinced that the way mankind can continue to raise itself up from our back-breaking labor and mud huts is through increasing our knowledge about the world we live in. And most important, he is convinced this knowledge is objective. We can find truth. It is verifiable. It can stand on its own.

In by far the largest "ecological" study of low-level radiation ever made, Professor Cohen was attempting to refine the Linear No-Threshold theory. But, in his words, "It came as a great shock to me that my data ran contrary to LNT, and I didn't fully believe it until about 1993—when I shut off the $1,200 radon reduction system in my home to save electricity." But he was using the **scientific method**, which is very clear about hypotheses that have been shown to be false: they are stuffed immediately into the trash can.

Under the LNT theory, cancer rate increases with increasing doses of radiation—*even at very low exposures.* If you are to plot response (cancer) versus dose, you should have a straight line with

---

[1] He mentions this in his terrific book, *The Nuclear Energy Option,* Plenum Press, New York, 1990, p. 269.

a positive slope according to this theory that has been sanctified by the regulators and rule writers. Using data from the American Academy of Sciences' Biological Effects of Ionizing Radiation committee (BEIR), the slope of this line should be an increased cancer risk of 4% per gray for chronic radiation and 8% per gray for acute exposure. By knowing the "whole body" dose given by various radon concentrations, this slope can also be expressed in terms of lung cancer mortality (since that is the only place in the body where significant radon progeny reside) per picocurie per liter of air. The value of this prediction for men, without any consideration of smoking, is 4.5 deaths per 10,000 men per year for each pCi/l increase in airborne radon. *Remember this figure.*

Cohen's initial study took five years, cost millions of dollars, and accumulated data from homes in 1,729 counties,[2] comprising about 90% of the U.S. population. It considered radon data from the EPA, state agencies, and 272,000 measurements made by the University of Pittsburgh. Census data on smoking, rural-urban balance, occupations, education, housing, medical care—a total of fifty-four socioeconomic "confounding" factors (alone and in combinations with each other) were analyzed to determine if and how they affected the lung cancer rate.

The study found—as you may now suspect—a discrepancy between the LNT's prediction of lung cancer and the actual data. This has since been known as "our discrepancy," and Cohen has invited his colleagues to try to find a confounder that would explain it. He notes that unless someone can come up with a reason to put aside "our discrepancy," the LNT must be considered a false and unacceptable theory and discarded as a source for use in regulatory authority. With more than 500 of the suspected confounders and combinations thereof already eliminated, it does not look good for the LNT advocates—most of whom do not address "our discrep-

---

[2] Because so many retirees move to California, Florida, and Arizona, these data were deleted, reducing the number of counties to 1,601. This deletion, incidentally, had an insignificant effect on the results.

Figure 33
Effect of Residential Radon Levels on Lung Cancer

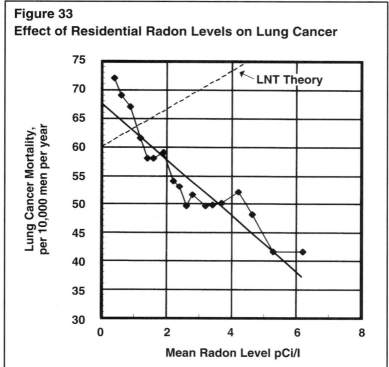

Note: Each data point represents an average of eighty-nine U.S. counties.

Source: Cohen, B.L. Test of the linear-no threshold theory of radiation carcinogenesis for inhaled radon decay products. *Health Physics,* 68, 157, 1995.

ancy" but prefer to snub Dr. Cohen as a mere physicist, and not an epidemiologist. (Critics overlook that G.A. Colditz is a world-class epidemiologist and was co-author with Cohen on "Tests of the linear-no-threshold theory for lung cancer induced by exposure to radon" in *Environmental Research,* 64, 1994.)

Figure 33 is typical of the curves plotted from the University of Pittsburgh data and is one of four similar figures in the report— this one is for males without smoking's being taken into account. The others are for males with smoking taken into consideration, and similar data on females both considering and not considering smoking.[3] I have deleted the error bars and the "first and third quartile" curves because I don't think they'd mean much to the average reader. Cohen also had indicators of the numbers of counties for each data point on his curves ranging from 4 to 216 with an average of 88.9. These are *counties,* bear in mind, not individuals.

Remember the increase by 4.5 deaths per pCi/l predicted by the LNT? That is shown graphically by the dashed line on Figure 33. The solid line with a *negative* slope is the best fit of the collected data. It shows a *minus* 4.7 deaths per pCi/l. If some hypothetical man (recall our graph is of male data) had a choice between being exposed to, say, 6 pCi of radon in his house, or being exposed to none, what is the significance of this choice? By sealing his house and spending some $3,000 to $4,000 for the government-recommended heat exchangers, he could *increase* his risk of lung cancer by 7.5%.

Perhaps that doesn't sound like much to you (especially if we're not talking about *your* lungs), but it is a huge increase in risk compared even with the LNTer's worst chortlings. You may recall the BEIR statistic for *chronic* radiation exposure predicts an increase in risk of cancer mortality of 8% for exposure to 2 gray, which is 200 cGy or 200,000 mrem. This is far above the risk experienced by all but a small fraction of A-bomb survivors! So if you missed Hiroshima and Nagasaki, just hang in there with the EPA recommendation on radon. They'll help you reach that goal of a significant increase in cancer risk!

I like the way Jay Lehr[4] summed up Cohen's results in an article, "Good News About Radon: The Linear Nonthreshold Model Is Wrong":

---

[3] These are available from his paper, "Test of the Linear-No-Threshold Theory of Radiation Carcinogenesis for Inhaled Radon Decay Products," *Health Physics,* February 1995. All curves give a similar negative correlation between radon and cancer through 6 pCi/l.

[4] Dr. Lehr is a senior scientist with Environmental Education Enterprises, a provider of high-technology short courses for environmental professionals.

Thus, in spite of extensive efforts to find a flaw in the obvious results indicated by the observed data, no potential explanation for the discrepancy between theory and reality could be found. It therefore appears that the linear no-threshold theory for carcinogenesis from inhaled radon decay products is invalid. This is indeed good news.

It would be even better news if more people knew about it.

Chapter 21
What's Cookin' in Those Reactors?

 *The use of thorium in CANDU type reactors would give earthlings sufficient energy to provide for the next seven ice ages.*
—Edward Teller[1]

EVIDENCE IN THE preceding chapters strongly indicates that hormetic stimulation from low levels of radiation has great potential for improving human health and vitality. For this to come about, we must be freed from the fears promoted by the Linear No-Threshold (LNT) theory and the principles of "collective dose."

Freedom from these unreasoned fears would also promote the growth of other nuclear technology, the most important of these probably being power generation. Availability of energy can be seen to coincide with both standard of living and heath. The environmental primitivists would have us live in a pristine wilderness—precisely where we see the absolute worst of the human condition. (And no McDonald's.)

Many of us would be interested in achieving greater independence from the utility companies (often government monopolies) and the government itself. We see all manner of solar toys and wind generators in *Mother Earth News,* which promise energy independence. Sure, as long as you have a staff of electrical and mechanical engineers, plus thousands of acres to mount the collectors or turbines, and a maintenance crew of dozens to keep things running. But as we shall see, nuclear energy has the promise to free those of us who would opt out of the government/utility networks. And while I take aim at some utilities that have become slovenly where licensure requirements have virtually eliminated competi-

---

[1] From "CANDU Is Really Remarkable," *Power Projections,* May, 1980.

tion, these same utilities would be in the best position to be the providers of community or residential power sources, having both generation and customer knowledge.

Mankind and Energy

The history of mankind is, in large part, a history of the harnessing of energy sources. Prehistoric man had only his own muscle power to wrest a livable habitat from his rugged environment. The discovery and control of fire eventually yielded metals, which improved the efficiency of muscle power and allowed the practical cultivation of crops. Domestication of animals—the horse, ox, donkey, elephant, dog—multiplied the energies of a man by severalfold. And this is where mankind remained for several thousand years.

While water wheels were used by several cultures for irrigation, the harnessing of hydropower was the product of the Industrial Revolution in mid-eighteenth-century England. The windmill was another attempt by man to increase his energy—one which is still going on, and still has the problem (as does hydropower) of requiring the cooperation of nature to utilize energy from the sun. (Both hydro and wind power are actually forms of solar energy, as are fossil fuels; but wood, coal, oil, and natural gas don't require quite as much cooperation from nature.)

Man's (and beasts') burden was lessened immeasurably by English engineer Thomas Savery who, in 1698, invented the "fire engine" to pump water from mines. Thomas Newcomen in 1705 and James Watt in 1763 improved the design to where the steam engine could be used for a variety of purposes, including transportation.

As the Industrial Revolution moved east to the continent, so did the desire for ways to deliver more energy—with less human and animal effort. Frenchman Jean Joseph Etienne Lenoir is credited with building the first gasoline internal combustion engine in 1860, while German Rudolf Diesel patented his engine in 1892 (and mysteriously disappeared from a London-bound German ship just prior to World War I.) The late nineteenth century saw the discovery and application of electrical principles by Dane Oersted, Frenchman Ampere, German Ohm, Englishman Faraday, American Henry, and Scotsman Maxwell—thus allowing energy to be transmitted from point of generation to point of need.

If we track both population and energy availability, we see that there has been a sixtyfold increase[2] in industrialized countries since Savery (compared with a world population that had been constant for a thousand years) and the same order of magnitude of energy usage *per capita*. But today, we have reached a plateau.

Enter the Atom

Let's return for a short graduate course from Hormesis U. about "splitting the atom."

We've already seen that U238[3] is an isotope of uranium with a half-life of 4.5 billion years. With a lump of this element and the proper instruments, you would find there is another isotope, U235, which amounts to only 0.7% of the total mass. Yet it is this tiny fraction that makes uranium the tremendous source of safe and reliable energy—not to mention the fearful master—that it has become.

U235,[4] like its more plentiful sibling, is an alpha emitter—but has a considerably shorter half-life…a mere 3,800,000 years, meaning that it was considerably more plentiful a billion or so years ago. It, along with plutonium 239 and U233, are the only isotopes that are **fissionable**—a phenomenon described below.

---

[2] Aren't you glad?—or there would be only a 1.6% chance that you would be here.

[3] I realize I said I was going to refer to isotopes in the form of ^{238}U or uranium 238. But U235 and U238 are such commonly used abbreviations to denote these isotopes that I will be using them in this chapter.

[4] U235 is sometimes referred to as "actinium" or "uranoactinium."

Under normal conditions, we can expect to see a U235 atom occasionally decay into an isotope of thorium and a helium nucleus (an alpha particle) similar to all radioactive isotopes experiencing *alpha decay*.[5] But let us suppose that a stray neutron smacks into the nucleus of an unsuspecting U235 atom. If the energy of the neutron is within a certain range, our U235 target atom *fissions*, that is, breaks into pieces.[6] It usually splits into two roughly equal parts, and most important, ejects about two neutrons. Obviously no atom could eject or emit *about* two neutrons, but, on average, that is what a fissioning U235 atom sends out of its nucleus.

Imagine, then, one of *these* neutrons hitting another U235 atom, which emits two neutrons with at least one of *these* splitting another atom…and so on, and so on. As you have no doubt already figured out, this is what is known as a **chain reaction**. When the ratio of fissioned atoms in successive generations is equal to one— that is, when one splitting atom causes exactly one more to split— the reaction is said to go **critical**. What happens to the other neutrons? They either escape from the volume of uranium, or they are absorbed—either unintentionally by structural material, or purposely by *control rods* made of boron, aluminum, cadmium, or several other neutron-absorbing materials—in order to keep the reaction under control (that is, to keep it from going **super-critical**). Does a super-critical reaction cause a bomb-like explosion? Not at all; if it did, bomb development by the Manhattan project would have been relatively simple rather than requiring the best theoretical physics minds on two continents. But super-criticality is no picnic. It causes rapid rises in fission reactions, leading to very

---

[5] "Occasionally" takes on a new meaning in the atomic world. Our roughly penny-sized gram of U235 would experience approximately 80,000 nuclear disintegrations per second.

[6] This was first observed by an unbelieving Lise Meitner in December 1938. She had observed barium, with an atomic number of 56, arising when she bombarded "actinium" with neutrons.

high temperatures that cause structural damage, torrents of neutrons, and "steam explosions." Bad, yes, but still light years away from the mushroom-shaped cloud.

Let's look at a few different types of reactors, with an eye for those that might allow decentralization of electric power generation.

Under the Grandstand

The first man-made chain reaction[7] occurred under the grandstand of the University of Chicago football field on December 2, 1942, in what was known as an atomic "pile." It was so named because it was constructed of a "pile" of 45,000 high-purity graphite bricks (250 tons), with 19,000 drilled holes to contain the approximately 93,000 pounds of uranium metal and uranium oxide along with the cadmium control rods. When operating at its design point, it generated a half watt of power—enough to almost power a pencil sharpener. (Fortunately, it was not designed as a power reactor, but as an experiment to prove the "chain reaction" hypothesis.)

Why the "high-purity graphite bricks"? It has to do with the statement a few paragraphs back about "…if the energy of the neutron is within a certain range." When we want to make little rocks out of big rocks, we are accustomed to using a bigger hammer and swinging harder. Not so in the nuclear world. In order for a neutron to have a decent chance at fissioning a U235 nucleus, it must be slowed down by the action of a **moderator**. Carbon—as long as it is of high enough purity to avoid absorbing the neutrons—is a good moderator, although, as Chernobyl demonstrated,

---

[7] There is much evidence that a natural reactor "happened" in Western Africa in the Republic of Gabon at Oklo some 1.7 billion years ago when the ratio of U235 to U238 was considerably higher. It appears to have operated in accordance with the Nuclear Regulatory Commission rules of that time and was safely shut down after several hundred thousand years of operation. See Oklo Reactor, *Scientific American,* August 1976.

it has a few potential problems—which is why U.S. power reactors *never* use this material...or this type of "graphite reactor." It is typically[8] used in military reactors for the production of plutonium—which reportedly was one of Chernobyl's functions, in addition to generating power.

Power Reactors

In the United States, power reactors are entirely of the PWR (pressurized water reactor) or the BWR (boiling water reactor) types. In both cases, water is used as the coolant *and* the moderator, which provides a very interesting advantage that probably no one has bothered to mention to you: If the coolant is lost, the chain reaction stops. Depending on the length of time the fuel has been producing power, the fuel rods may or may not be thermally and radioactively "hot" from the *daughters* of the fissioning process. Even in the worst case, the heat generated is no more than 1% or 2% of that during normal operation. This is why the "disaster" at Three Mile Island didn't really happen—except in the minds of the uninformed.

While the Japanese installed the first Advanced Boiling Water Reactor (ABWR) in 1996, none of the new, modular designs have seen the light of day in this country. Not only have we been blinded by the *non-threat* of low-level radiation, but the cost of building a nuclear plant has escalated by a factor of seventeen, after considering inflation—mostly from construction delays caused by environmentalist lawsuits. (The above-mentioned Japanese ABSR plant took fifty-two months to build—compared with more than eleven years for the most recent plant in the United States.) I *would* say the new designs are even safer than the old—but how do you get safer than no deaths, no injuries, and no negative effects to the public

---

[8] Other uses would be in research reactors, as well as in reactors for use in creating medical radionuclides.

from several thousand reactor years of operation with thousands of gigawatt-hours of life-enhancing electrical energy having been generated?[9] Nonetheless, neither the PWR or BWR has much promise for miniaturization and "local" use as—by nature—they operate with high-power densities, which have the potential to cause a messy and expensive loss-of-coolant accident. They also require pumps, back-up pumps, and relatively elaborate controls.

All of these U.S. power reactors use **enriched** uranium as a fuel, as do reactors in France (where 80% of the electrical power comes from nuclear energy), Japan, England, and most other countries. The enrichment process starts with natural uranium, which is dissolved in acid to produce uranium hexafluoride gas. This ultra-corrosive gas is then pumped thousands of times through membranes where the lighter U235 passes through just a little bit easier than the U238. For power reactors, the U235 is enriched from 0.7% to about 3.5%,[10] which takes not only lots of time but considerable energy.

CANDU and SLOWPOKE

While the United States—with its post–World War II enrichment technology and capacity—built power reactors using enriched uranium, the Canadians took a different approach. You may recall that deuterium (^2H) reacts with oxygen to form "heavy water"—an unusually good moderator that bounces back and slows down neutrons that might ordinarily escape the reactor. The most interesting thing about the Canadian CANDU heavy water reactor—from the standpoint of community or home power plants—is

---

[9] Some of the media scream "disaster" when ten gallons of water with $^1/80$ the radioactivity of salad oil leak out in the process of heating and otherwise providing life-giving energy to an entire city. Why doesn't it make front-page news when some one falls off the roof to his death trying to clean the solar collector—which provides a few puny kilowatts of solar energy for warming the hot water...when the sun is shining?

[10] "Bomb grade" U235 must be enriched to 90%—an extremely difficult process. (Thank goodness, or any crackpot might be able to do it.)

that it uses natural (unenriched) uranium. This doesn't get them off the hook from an initial energy expenditure, however, since heavy water is expensive to separate—about $100 per pound and costing $100 million dollars for a full-scale 1,000 megawatt reactor. It does, however, eliminate the problem of enrichment. The CANDU design has many parallel fuel assemblies with the heavy water coolant/moderator flowing through each. To refuel the reactor, it doesn't need to be shut down; you just cut off the water to stop the nuclear reaction in a section isolated for refueling, and then change out the "spent" fuel assemblies.[11]

Even more interesting from the standpoint of decentralization is the Canadian SLOWPOKE[12] reactor, which is as safe and secure as a Sierra Club official working for the Environmental Protection Agency. Figure 34 shows a cutaway sketch of this "pool" type reactor—so named because it operates submerged in a pool of water. Unlike PWRs and BWRs, it does not have "defense in depth"—because it doesn't need it. The laws of physics provide it with more than enough protection.

The original design[13] has a maximum operating temperature of 80°C with a cylindrical core about nine inches in diameter by nine inches in height. Surrounding the enriched-uranium fuel assembly are beryllium reflectors, which keep the reactor *critical* … as long as the water density remains high. If the reactor "heats up," the lower water density slows the reaction bringing the temperature back to the design point.

---

[11] "Spent" fuel assemblies aren't really spent at all—they have more than 95% of the initial fuel remaining with only a few percent of "daughters" that contaminate the rest and absorb the needed neutrons.

[12] Safe LOW POwer Kritical Experiment—but it's not experimental anymore, having been in operation for more than twenty-five years. (Canadians may be great reactor designers, but they seem to have a little problem with their spelling.)

[13] SLOWPOKE I and II have been operational for some time; the series is now up to V or VI but I haven't been able to get much information on the later models.

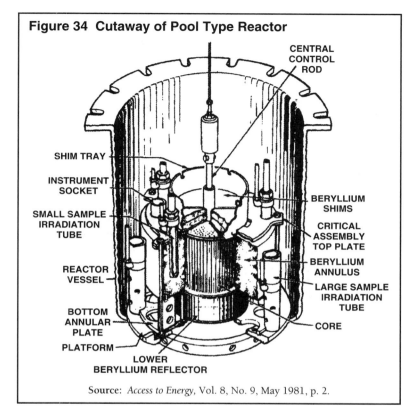

Figure 34 Cutaway of Pool Type Reactor

CENTRAL CONTROL ROD

SHIM TRAY

INSTRUMENT SOCKET

SMALL SAMPLE IRRADIATION TUBE

REACTOR VESSEL

BOTTOM ANNULAR PLATE

PLATFORM

LOWER BERYLLIUM REFLECTOR

BERYLLIUM SHIMS

CRITICAL ASSEMBLY TOP PLATE

BERYLLIUM ANNULUS

LARGE SAMPLE IRRADIATION TUBE

CORE

Source: *Access to Energy,* Vol. 8, No. 9, May 1981, p. 2.

Suppose all the water evaporates or is sloshed out by an earth-quake? Naturally, the reaction stops, as the moderator is gone. But also the power density is so low that nothing happens to the fuel. The reactor just goes dormant until someone takes an action to bring it back to life.[14] As Canadian scientist Dr. John Hilborn, who conducted experiments leading to the SLOWPOKE, said, "It is safer without operators than with them."[15]

The original SLOWPOKEs were not designed as power reac-tors. Their heat output (which is considerably higher than any

---

[14] Typically the operators do not have access to the reactor.

[15] From an interview with Petr Beckmann, *Access to Energy,* Vol.8, No.9, May 1981, pp. 1–2.

possible electrical output) is a mere twenty kilowatts, equivalent to about thirteen hair dryers. Their function, as mentioned, was not to produce electricity but to transmute certain materials into radionuclides, primarily for medical purposes. But the concept of a low-temperature, inherently safe, non-polluting, inexpensive-to-fuel, produce-power-where-you-need-it reactor is intriguing for those who would like to have energy independence.[16]

SECURE and the IFR

Other low-temperature reactors—used for warming entire communities—are not new to the world...just to U.S. citizens with our abysmal lack of scientific knowledge. For instance, a Swedish and Finnish consortium has designed a 200 MW inherently safe reactor called SECURE[17] —with no moving parts, not even control rods— as the reactivity level is controlled by the content of boric acid in the coolant/moderator.

Finally, there is another reactor design known as the Integral Fast Reactor,[18] which I find fascinating, because it is fueled by natural uranium and is as close to a perpetual motion machine as we are likely to get. It operates in a vessel filled with liquid sodium (melting point, 208°F), which is a much better heat-transfer agent than water—along with having certain desirable nuclear characteristics. It reportedly produces 100 to 200 times more electrical energy per pound of fuel than obtainable from existing plants. The prototype plant, at Idaho Falls, was designed to be virtually self-contained with the capability of fabricating, using, and reprocessing the spent fuel "on-site." It is inherently safe from a meltdown, since the fuel assemblies are configured in such a manner as to shut

---

[16] Some electric utilities might oppose such a competitive concept, but they would, as mentioned, be in the best position to provide service for local power reactors.

[17] Safe and Environmentally Clean Urban REactor

[18] See *Integral Fast Reactor,* available from Argonne National Laboratories, P.O. Box 2528, Idaho Falls, ID 83415.

down the reaction when the temperature increases above its maximum design point. As a test, the entire heat transfer system was shut down while operating at full power—without causing any harm to the reactor.

While it is unlikely that the fuel-processing part of the operation could be scaled down to community or residential proportions, the inherent safety of the reactor is intriguing, along with its use of natural (unenriched) uranium. It is likely that radiation would be an insignificant factor compared with keeping the sodium contained, since contact with either water or air causes some pretty nasty chemical reactions. (It is best kept submerged in kerosene or naphtha.)

As far as I know, a low-power, inherently safe reactor has not been designed for community or home use. Why? I suspect it's because the prevailing fear of low-level radiation would keep any reasonably intelligent investor in the "sow bellies futures" market where at least there is a chance of making a profit. Why design a product that will cost more in attorneys' fees each time you sell one than the sale price of the product itself? Although much of the technology is there and proven, it just won't happen in today's climate ruled by the Linear No-Threshold bureaucracy.

But if we can create an understanding of *actual*—as opposed to perceived—radiation dangers, the technology will surely flourish. Because of higher efficiencies? No, large power reactors operating at high temperatures have higher efficiencies than would a home or community reactor and are well suited for commercial and industrial power production—but they also have transmission losses, transformer losses, costs of installing and maintaining pole-line hardware, and other overhead expenses that can be eliminated by decentralization, especially for small, off-the-beaten-path residential customers who use only a few thousand kilowatt-hours per month.

Would we require a government program to make this happen? Not at all. Just get the government out of the way, and let market forces determine what is worthy and what is not. As Paul Johnson put it,

> For capitalism merely occurs, if no one does anything to stop it. It is socialism that has to be constructed, and as a rule, forcibly imposed, thus providing a far bigger role for intellectuals in its genesis.[19]

---

[19] "The heartless lovers of humankind," *Wall Street Journal,* January 5, 1987.

Chapter 22
Energy: Don't Leave Home Without It

Did we miss the "nuclear vehicle" boat because of our fears and the rules imposed on the nuclear industry? "What might have been" is truly an impossible question to answer.

WITH THE POPULATION of the Earth now surpassing 6 billion, and the requirement for energy *per capita* continually increasing as mankind is being liberated from the yoke, we can expect an exponential increase in the requirement for energy. Some of you believe that we need to limit the population of the world. I disagree—and if you're interested you can read a summary of my position in the footnote.[1] Some would fear that our unspoiled wilderness and irreplaceable wildlife will be destroyed if the population continues to grow. Again, I disagree, but go to the footnote only if this is of any interest to you.[2] Regardless of what you *believe,* the odds are in favor of a continued growth with these trends predominating. So what are to be the energy sources in the future?

Many environmentalists are excited about solar power. How can you blame them? It's everywhere—and it's free. But there are a

---

[1] In the thousands of years that the Earth had a low and "flat" population, the inhabitants suffered unbelievable deprivation by our standards. Today the population of the Earth *and* the standard of living are higher than ever. An unproductive person is indeed a drain on society; but, until government prevents it, more people are in productive activities than living off the productive.

[2] If you want to see true environmental catastrophe, take a look at (a) the energy-impoverished countries where vegetation is stripped to the roots as a source of cooking fuel and tribesman must spend most of their day's energy output in foraging for firewood, or (b) the Eastern-bloc countries, where almost an entire continent would be declared a Superfund site under our system. And you might note that only those creatures that are "owned by all of us" are in danger. Species in private hands do quite well.

few other considerations. While many low-powered applications, are feasible, when it comes down to *commercial and industrial* applications, solar energy becomes pretty darn environmentally hostile. A fairly modest eight- or nine-story suburban office building might require a megawatt of electrical energy at its peak monthly need. The dedicated solar energy plant—with 10% efficiency (not yet attainable), a 50% collector spacing, and a load factor of 75% (it must be able to supply 75% of the maximum load at any time)— required to support this building situated on less than one acre of ground, would need approximately 100 to 300 acres of collection and storage (battery) space, depending on climate. Energy-intensive industrial plants could easily require 500 to 1,000 acres of solar facility for each factory acre. Just as it would be a lovely thing to have a solar-powered car like those that race on the Australian desert (in the daytime), it is just a crying shame that the sun doesn't supply more than one kilowatt per square meter anywhere on Earth.

Wind energy has such obvious problems with availability—in addition to being very insensitive to passing birds and eerily noisy to nearby residents—that it really can't qualify as a reliable source. And while hydroelectric power is a wonderful thing (until the dam silts up), there are only a limited number of sites in the United States with any real energy potential. Imagine, if you will, trying to build a hydroelectric dam in Florida or southern Louisiana, and you'll get the idea. I'm not even going to discuss chicken manure or geothermal energy. If you're hanging your hat on these, you're obviously in the wrong book.

The Cornucopia of Nuclear Power

You will remember from chapter 21 that we have two neutrons, on average, emitted whenever a U235 atom undergoes fission—or "splitting." One of these is necessary to fission another atom to keep the chain reaction going. But what happens to all of those second neutrons? Some of them, as mentioned, are absorbed by the structure of the reactor or by the control rods, which slide in and out of the reactor to keep the reaction at—or just very slightly above—the *critical* point. But others smash into, and are captured by, the plentiful U238 atoms that make up from 95% to 96.5% of the fuel rod contents. When this happens, a truly miraculous thing takes place: This practically worthless material is transformed into one of the most concentrated sources of energy on Earth—or in the universe for that matter—plutonium 239, an element so evil that it was named for the god of the underworld. (Not really, but that's what some would have you believe.)[3] This happens in every one of the world's 500 power reactors, plus thousands of research reactors, every day they are in operation. In fact, a sizable fraction (up to about 30%) of electrical energy generated by a power plant comes from this plutonium, which arises as a natural consequence of the uranium fission reaction—without any effort on our part—and supplements the scarce U235 fuel.

Some reactors, however, are designed to intentionally make plutonium. If it is to be used in bombs, it is normally made in a reactor with another modulator—such as the carbon-modulated reactor at Chernobyl. A reactor designed specifically to make only fuel-grade plutonium is called a **breeder reactor**, since new fuel is "bred" from an almost worthless byproduct of the refining cycle.[4] Are we speculating here on new technology like "fusion" power? Hardly.

The first reactor ever to produce electric power from nuclear energy was a "liquid metal fast breeder reactor" known as the EBR-I. (By the way, *liquid metal* means that the coolant was not our old friend water, but liquid sodium; *fast* means that it used "fast

---

[3] Plutonium was named in honor of the discovery of the planet Pluto, just as neptunium and uranium were named for Neptune and Uranus.

[4] Breeder technology *seems* to be on hold for a couple of reasons: (1) in the prevailing anti-nuclear climate, few entrepreneurs or speculators are willing to make investments in nuclear power for fear of laws that can make their investments instantly worthless; and (2) at the present time there is a glut of plutonium available from the dismantlement of nuclear weapons.

neutrons," not the slowed-down, moderated variety.) Designed by physicist Walter Zinn in 1944, his brainchild went *critical* at 11 A.M., December 20, 1951—producing the first steam in history produced by man-made nuclear heat. Like the Manhattan reactor in Chicago and the SLOWPOKE reactor in Canada, EBR-I[5] was not designed to produce electrical power but to prove the concept of fuel breeding (which it did along with its successor, EBR-II). The EBR-II had "on the spot reprocessing," which reprocessed 35,000 fuel elements between 1965 and 1969. But the facility was not without problems: the fence around it kept out the coyotes, causing the rabbit population to outbreed the reactor.

Does the EBR-II sound a little familiar? It should since it has another name we used in chapter 21—the Integral Fast Reactor (IFR).

While many U.S. politicians have never heard of breeder technology, Europeans have. Sadly, "Green" activists there have been successful in shutting them down or keeping them from ever starting up.

Five Million Miles on a Pound of Plutonium?

In the early 1950s, when I was an almost-teenager reading all the popular magazines on science and mechanics I could read at the drugstore newsstand, there were articles on "atomic propulsion" for every conceivable vehicle from motorcycles to space ships. (Well, maybe not motorcycles.) A lot of the concepts were just that: concepts. Grandiose ideas sold magazines but would probably not have done much to power your fishing boat.

Only a few years later we learned the horrors of exposure to radiation. I can remember reading—even before age thirteen—not only the heart-rending stories of A-bomb victims, but also about

---

[3] Declared a national landmark in 1966, the EBR-1 is open to the public from mid June to mid September. Located eighteen miles southeast of Arco, Idaho, on Highway 26, visitors must be at least sixteen years old (too much neutron violence?) and U.S. citizens (fear of spies who might steal this technology?).

the unfortunate Japanese fishermen who were accidentally exposed to H-bomb test fall-out. I thought they all had died. (Although billed by the press as "Lethally Exposed," except for the one who died from acute radiation sickness, none of the other twenty-two was a cancer fatality as of twenty-five years after exposure.)[6]

It wasn't long after this that the "atomic power" articles, and much of the interest in nuclear technology, dried up. The Linear No-Threshold hypothesis was soon to send all of those ideas into the black hole of radiation avoidance—which later became radiation hysteria. Did we miss the "nuclear vehicle" boat because of our fears and the rules imposed on the nuclear industry? "What might have been" is truly an impossible question to answer. Thousands of independently acting entrepreneurs *would* have answered it for us, had they been given the chance.

Neither the pressurized water reactor (PWR) nor the boiling water reactor (BWR)—the mainstays of the U.S. nuclear power industry—are adaptable to smaller scale, mobile applications. A variation of the CANDU reactor principle would come closer by using low-boiling-point compounds such as CFCs to spin a turbine, but even that is a stretch for anything smaller than a large bus. (Not to say that it couldn't be done if technology is given a chance.)

But why worry about atomic-powered anythings? What we're currently using is working out pretty well, isn't it? True, but let's look for a moment at how we fuel our vehicles. And though I don't think we are in danger of "running out of oil" any time soon, it is logical to assume that the energy cost of obtaining oil will increase as the oil-bearing strata become more and more difficult to access.

---

[6] Kumatori, T., Ishihara, T., Hirshima, K. Sugiyama, H., Ishii, S., and Miyoshi, K.. Follow-up studies over a twenty-five-year period on the Japanese fishermen exposed to radioactive fallout in 1954. *The Medical Basis for Radiation Preparedness,* Hubner, K.F., and Fry, A. A., editors, Elsevier, New York, 1980.

If we take your politically incorrect sports utility vehicle out on the open road with one pound of gasoline in it, the heat energy content of the fuel will propel you about three miles. By comparison the heat energy in one pound of plutonium would take you some 5,420,000 miles down the road—using the same efficiency figure as the gasoline engine.[7] Since this is about thirty times more than the typical mechanical life of a vehicle, it is likely that any nuclear-powered vehicle would be fueled for life at the factory.

All well and good, you might say. But what about the lack of adaptability of power-plant technology to mobile vehicles? Good question. There are other nuclear technologies, besides trying to shrink a power plant, that would be interesting to explore. One of these is the **radioisotope thermo-electric generator** or RTG.

The RTG is based on a very simple[8] physical principle known as thermoelectricity. If you take two wires of different materials and connect their junctions in a loop, a current will flow when the temperature of the "hot junction" is greater than that of the "cold junction." In the RTG, a radioisotope supplies the heat, while a "heat sink"—such as you might find on the rear of a high-powered stereo amplifier—cools the cold junction. Any number of junctions can be connected in series (known as a **thermopile**) to produce whatever voltage is desired, while connections are paralleled to increase the current flow. The inherent low voltage of the device can be increased with a dc-to-dc or dc-to-ac converter.[9] An obvious

---

[7] The efficiency would be lower using today's technology. But even at half or a quarter the already-low efficiencies of internal combustion engines, the incredible heat content of many radioactive isotopes makes for unbelievable comparisons to all fossil fuels.

[8] "Simple" in practice, as anyone can connect different types of wires together; the theory, known as the *Seebeck effect,* is a little more complicated.

[9] Transformers, used on alternating current circuits, do not work for direct current. A "dc-to-dc" converter *chops* the dc, making it appear to be ac, transforms it to a different voltage, and then rectifies it back to dc.

advantage of the thermo-electric generator is its total lack of moving parts—since electrons don't count.

The Manhattan project scientists had inadvertently discovered this "warmness" of the plutonium 239 isotope.[10] Project experimenters supposedly used the plutonium received from the Hanford reservation—gleaned and refined at an almost unbelievable price—as hand warmers. While alpha particles lose their energy too quickly to penetrate the skin, these atomic "shot-puts" collide with and agitate atoms with which they come in contact, hence the feeling of warmth.

As we might expect, the rate of decay of the isotope has much to do with an isotope's heat-producing potential. While bomb-grade plutonium 239 (with its 24,110-year half-life) is okay for hand warmers, another plutonium isotope (atomic weight 238, with a half-life of only 87.7 years) is the candidate of choice for our extraterrestrial deep-space probes. Plutonium 238 can *really* kick atoms around, to *way* beyond the boiling point of water.[11]

This is not new technology. All deep-space probes *must* have some sort of nuclear power supply, as none of the alternatives are able to supply usable amounts of power for the years it takes to complete these missions. Batteries are out of the question for even short missions, and solar panels don't work well, since the energy available drops off as the square of the distance from the sun. A ten-by-ten-foot collector for Earth-Moon operations, for instance, would swell to tennis court size for missions to Jupiter, and blossom to the equivalent of more than two football fields for exploration of Neptune. Moreover, Earth-based solar cells are not easy to mount efficiently, even with a solid *terra firma* foundation. How about

---

[10] Actually all radioactive isotopes generate heat as a byproduct of decay—but both the rate and the type of decay emissions are important. You really wouldn't want to cozy up with a strong gamma ray emitter.

[11] Spacecraft power supplies operate at approximately 800°F. RTG temperatures can exceed 1300°F.

trying to maneuver football-field sized collector banks—structures and deployment mechanisms—in a zero-gravity environment?[12]

While the RTG has been the only practical choice for deep-space missions, anti-nuclear propagandists have portrayed it as a hazard to the entire human race because of its use of plutonium fuel. The misguided protesters wring their hands over seventy-two pounds of plutonium that they contend might somehow be released into the atmosphere and over the effect that might have on humankind. However, they *totally ignore* the fact that two to three *tons* of various vaporized (and hence, breathable) plutonium isotopes were injected into the biosphere by the Nagasaki bomb and the hundreds of above-ground tests just after World War II; yet the last time I looked, the human race was still alive and kicking.

While spacecraft have shown the reliability and longevity of the RTG, why haven't there been applications in transportation utilizing this technology?[13] It certainly doesn't require a rocket scientist to conceive of an RTG automobile that would have both a generator and auxiliary batteries available for acceleration and hills—yet would recharge itself, both while driving and while sitting all day in a parking lot. But if you remember the story about the Goianians, you may have already considered the possibility of being stoned

---

[12] Fuel cells would be fine, except that the weight of the fuel—and its containers—wouldn't allow for much else on the voyage. We might want to note, thanks to the science education given by the mission and movie *Apollo 13*, most of us are now well aware that fuel cells must carry their own oxidizer—which, in the case of oxygen, was not readily available in interlunar space.

[13] Another very successful use of the plutonium RTG was in pacemakers. From 1973 through 1987, 155 radioisotope-powered pacemakers were implanted in a Newark Beth Israel Medical Center study. With a half-life of eighty-seven years, the nuclear devices outlasted battery operated devices—which required surgery for re-implantation—by many years and were ultra-reliable. And although "it has been shown beyond any reasonable doubt that there is no increased risk of malignancy in this group of patients" few, if any, new nuclear devices are being installed. Why? It's our good friend, the Linear No-Threshold hypothesis. See "The Nuclear Pacemaker: Is Renewed Interest Warranted?" *American Journal of Cardiology*, Oct. 1990.

whenever you pulled your Plutoniumobile out of the garage—not to mention having to deal with swarms of bureaucrats from every imaginable protective agency who would be on the spot to make sure no stray alpha ray is loosed on the public. With incentives like these for the buyer, entrepreneurs are not exactly standing in line to enter this market.

Want to get 5,420,000 miles to the pound? Me too. Sorry to say that's never going to happen, because the long-standing and difficult problem of squeezing *actual* energy from *potential* energy is fraught with some inconvenient impossibilities. But if we are to *approach* the theoretical limits of physical science, it will take an understanding of the *real* dangers of radiation, and getting the government out of the policing business. Plus, no doubt, many billions of dollars in research and development costs; but that's what capitalists do: invest their money to make profits from producing things that cause our lives to be more satisfying.

Oh, and not to worry. Manufacturers of nuclear-powered vehicles are not going to fry their customers with gamma rays any more than Campbell's would put botulin toxin in the soup.

It's not good for business.

But What About Fusion?

It is so inviting…to think that our planet can be powered from ocean water. *That,* as you probably well know, is the expectation of many who would eschew other forms of energy generation. "Cold fusion"—which many of us would *hope* to be a viable energy source—is unproven. Which leads, naturally, to the hot variety. And I do mean hot!

You may remember from your freshman days at Hormesis U., that both deuterium and tritium are isotopes of hydrogen. (See chapter 5 if your memory is a bit rusty.) As it is generally understood, a fusion reaction in the sun occurs at temperatures in excess of 1,000,000°F, when a deuterium and a tritium atom are crushed together to form helium and expel a neutron. It would be much cleaner if two deuterium atoms could do the trick without a neutron chaperone, but the universe just wasn't made that way. And while it's true that there is a virtually infinite supply of deuterium in ocean water, the horrible fact is: there isn't any tritium. (OK, a few quadrillion atoms or so, but not any that we can extract.) In fact, in the entire United States, there isn't much tritium at all, since your government considers this beta emitter— used on luminous watch dials—to be hazardous to your life. (Please be appreciative.)

Where would we get the tritium? I don't know, and I don't think anyone else does either. But there are other problems that I suspect are overwhelming in light of our present-day engineering and material capabilities—and may be physically impossible to solve.[14] First, the energy required to magnetically contain the process (the only way it can be contained, since these temperatures decompose all materials into constituent atoms) invariably requires more energy than can be generated. Yet if, and when, this obstacle can be overcome, we have the problem of that pesky neutron.

While other particles can be redirected magnetically to where they have little danger to humans or equipment, the electrically neutral neutron has a mind of its own. When a plethora of neutrons are released around normal materials, those materials are transmuted into other elements that are typically radioactive. Wouldn't this make the fusion reactor radioactive? Yes it would, which is probably why hot-fusion experiments reportedly must be cooled-down, dismantled, and decontaminated after every test run of only a few seconds. This might prompt us to ask, "What about the delivery of energy, twenty-four hours per day, 365 days per year?" There are, in my opinion, two choices.

---

[14] For more on this subject, see the August 1999 edition of *The Energy Advocate*, published by Howard Hayden, professor emeritus of Physics, University of Connecticut. P.O. Box 7595, Pueblo West, CO 81007—or www.EnergyAdvocate.com. ($35/year.)

Energy Sources for the Future—Take Your (Limited) Choice(s)

Fossil fuels will be around as long as mankind, but there is historical reason to believe that they—like whale oil and placer gold—will be diminishing in economically recoverable supplies. "Renewable resources"—such as solar, wind, hydro, tidal, geothermal, and chicken manure energies—are frankly just not going to fill the bill when it comes to an industrial economy with billions of people requiring an ever-increasing supply of energy.[15] Fusion, as noted, would be wonderful...if it is possible as a source, and if we have the ability to develop it in the next twenty generations. Which leaves us with one proven source of sufficient energy for the world during the next several millennia: nuclear fission. There are, as far as is known today—and we know quite a bit—only three choices for fissionable materials.

Number 1: Uranium 235. This is the granddad of fission. It naturally occurs as 0.7% of the element found on Earth, and—if economically recoverable supplies are considered—is probably good for powering the world's energy needs for the next century or so. Many observers say forty years, but "Julian Simon's Law"[16] would no doubt govern this commodity also.

Number 2: Plutonium 239. Easily "bred" from common uranium 238, transmutation of existing stockpiles should last several hundred years at present use rates. But as Dr. Cohen points out in *The Nuclear Energy Option*, with breeder technology it becomes economical to separate uranium from sea water—where there are some 2 trillion curies—allowing man all the energy he needs until the sun burns out in 4 or 5 billion years.

Number 3: Uranium 233. This is the sleeper. When thorium 232 is exposed to neutrons, as in the transmutation of U238 to Pu239, another miraculous thing happens. Dirt becomes an incredible

---

[15] For instance, energy-balance calculations reveal that the energy cost of building a solar plant exceeds the energy it is expected to capture and utilize over a forty-year lifetime.

[16] Simon, Julian. *The Ultimate Resource,* Princeton University Press, Princeton, 1996.

energy source. As mentioned in chapter 1, the Earth's surface averages 2.5 tons of thorium in the first foot of each square mile of area. The late Dr. Edward Teller[17] was a strong advocate of thorium transmutation using a CANDU-type heavy-water reactor. His design would allow plentiful and inexpensive thorium to be entered in one side of the reactor, converted slowly to U233, which would be fissioned for power, with the "really spent" fuel exiting from the other side months or years later. He calculates this would give earthlings sufficient energy to provide for the next seven ice ages.[18]

Add this to Dr. Cohen's four or five billion years, and we're really starting to talk about some time.

What's the Holdup?

Fuel reprocessing and breeder reactors are major world-class technologies that our government is keeping its citizens and non-international businesses from participating in. Without it, the fuel for our existing reactors is in jeopardy of becoming uneconomical to mine and process within the next several decades. And without it, we as a nation will be starved for energy *and* uncompetitive in the world marketplace. How can this be? Who would stifle the production and distribution of energy? Who would not stem the misery brought about by an energy poverty?

I am sad to say, there are those who seek this condition. I don't think they believe themselves hateful or misanthropic. They feel that *sacrificing others* today will bring about a better life for many more *others*. They are the spiritual descendants of Thomas Malthus and Ned Ludd—and are not aware of the vast gains of the industrial revolution in general, and nuclear power in particular. Nor are they

---

[17] Known as the "Father of the H-bomb"—but more accurately described as the defender of the free world from Soviet totalitarianism.

[18] From "CANDU Is Really Remarkable," *Power Projections*, May 1980.

aware of the ability of markets to provide a life with great worth for billions of participants and critics alike.

I feel sorry for them in their lack of knowledge.

And Finally…

Many of us think in terms of our present energy situation and don't consider what benefits our world would have if the LNT did not cloud the minds of those who could do great works—if allowed to do so by the regulators. While the American Nuclear Society is still on the fence in regard to scrapping the LNT and recognizing the possibilities of hormesis, Gregg M. Taylor, the editor-in-chief of the organization's magazine—*Nuclear News*—wrote an absorbing editorial entitled, "We have met the solution, and it is us."

In this monograph, he noted that one of California's big problems—echoed in many countries around the world—is the availability of water for agricultural irrigation. Water from the Colorado River is coveted by all and is a constant source of political turmoil. But what if we built nuclear desalination plants, he asks, strategically located along the coast? They could be pollution free—with guppy rights properly observed.

One might wonder how this could dovetail into Dr. Cohen's extraction of uranium from the sea—surely there is a synergistic connection here as part of the desalination process could well be the initial step in obtaining the metal. How much more habitable—for people like you and me—would the Earth become if our deserts could be irrigated…at no cost *except the premature use of the nuclear energy in uranium and thorium.* They are going to lose their energy over time anyway—we're just appropriating it for our short-term use. Besides, a quarter of the uranium and two-thirds of the thorium would still have its energy when the sun flakes out on us in eight or ten billion years.

Editor Taylor also touches on another touchy subject: toxic wastes. Noting that most of us remember "disintegrators" from our sci-fi days, he observes that it takes only sufficient energy—which can be provided readily by clean nuclear sources—to reduce the most horrible kinds of toxic waste into its constituent atoms, which would totally lose their identity and could be recombined as the purest substances possible.

Let your mind roam free for a moment. What scourge of mankind might not be alleviated by sufficient energy availability?

• Floods and hurricanes? Better materials requiring more energy, higher dikes—both a function of available energy

• Starvation? Hydroponics from desalinated water

• Locusts? Airplanes, chemicals, huge nuclear flyswatters (just kidding).

*　*　*　*　*

If man is to advance to another higher plateau—past the industrial and information revolutions—it can be done only in conjunction with an unencumbered access to energy. Otherwise, we are dooming generations to untold misery and suffering.

Chapter 23
The Dirty Bomb's Dirty Little Secret

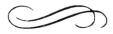 *Anyone who has the slightest familiarity with nuclear power knows that it is impossible to steal fuel from an operating reactor.*

Is THERE A nuclear threat to Western civilization? No question. As long as there are nuclear weapons and Islamic terrorists who would murder thousands of innocents without conscience, such a possibility exists. Actions to prevent this are a subject far afield from hormesis, but one possibility might be to offer a higher-than-market price for plutonium to be blended into MOX,[1] rendering it unusable for weapons, as a fuel for power reactors.

Dirty Bombs

We have been led to believe—on the basis of the LNT theory and collective dose—that terrorists could mount an effective attack by the use of "dirty bombs," i.e., bombs that spread radioactive materials by use of conventional explosives. At present, such bombs would be an effective weapon, since the fear of radiation, as in Goia and Three Mile Island, would doubtlessly cause panic and result in deaths from heart attacks, auto accidents, and the like. But if we understand the actual effects of radiation, we can respect it without allowing it to overcome our rational thought. Let's look at the worst case.

Terrorists park a car bomb filled with strontium 90, which has a long half-life (twenty-nine years) and the propensity for replacing

---

[1] MOX is mixed oxide fuel composed of 7% plutonium mixed with depleted uranium. Currently about 2% of reactor fuel is MOX. A very good discussion of MOX and the use of reactor-grade plutonium in weapons can be found online at the following address: www.nic.com.au/nip42.htm

calcium in bones. At noon, with the maximum number of people walking down Wall Street on the way to lunch, the bomb is exploded, and strontium 90 is blasted into the air. Radioactive debris is scattered by the wind over an area of many blocks.

Let's look at this scenario as graduates of Hormesis U. First, where are terrorists going to get a carload of strontium 90? It is a product of nuclear explosions and found in reactor "wastes." Like so many other "waste" radionuclides, it is a valuable commodity being used in medical and agricultural tracers as well as in RTGs (radio thermo-electric generators) for navigational beacons and weather stations. Medically, it is used for treatment of eye diseases and bone cancer. It is a valuable commodity and certainly not widely available in quantities like the ammonium nitrate and fuel oil used in the Oklahoma City bombing.

The EPA's Radiation Information website[2] tells us that "swallowing Sr-90 with food or water is the primary pathway of intake."

The same source tells us that strontium 90 is a beta emitter. Graduates of Hormesis U. know that beta radiation can travel only a few feet through air and causes minor burns (beta burns) to exposed skin. Knowing this, what action would be required after a terrorist went to the trouble and expense to disburse this most dreaded of radioactive materials in the canyons of Manhattan? I would suggest a warning to the local inhabitants not to lick the pavement or buildings. After that, I would wait for a rain that would wash the dust down the sewers leading to the Atlantic Ocean, where there are already quadrillions of curies (septillions of becquerels) that will still be there long after the vestiges of strontium 90 have disappeared. A potential problem: the sewer rats might be affected bio-positively and take charge of the large metropolitan cities.

So much for dirty bombs.

---

[2] www.epa.gov/radiation/radionuclides/strontium.htm

Where the Terrorists Have Already Won

In 1978, Jimmy Carter reneged on the opening of a reprocessing plant that was nearing completion in Barnwell, South Carolina. This facility was to take "spent" fuel rods from power reactors owned by the utilities, dissolve them in acid, then separate the uranium and plutonium from the contaminants that would "poison" and eventually stop the chain reaction. The highly radioactive *progeny* of the energy-producing reactions—amounting to some 1% or 2% of the volume—would be disposed of by any one of a number of perfectly safe methods. The fuel portion would then be reformed into uranium or "MOX" pellets for insertion into fuel assemblies.

Hold on. Could one infer from this that these "spent" fuel elements contain in excess of 95% of their initial fuel? Yes, one could. Is *this* what we plan to bury under Yucca Mountain? Precisely.

Does this make sense to you? It certainly doesn't to the English, French, Japanese, Russians, and others who think we are absolutely *nuts* for planning to bury unbelievable amounts of readily obtainable energy. But it made sense to the Carter administration, and even though Reagan reversed the decision, there were no corporate takers who were willing to risk their shareholders' money on a project that could be changed by the whim of a government with a history of caving in to the slightest pseudo-environmentalist pressure. And there would certainly be pressure—since, as we "know," *all* radiation is dangerous, since any gamma ray could cause cancer…even though the odds against it are 30 quadrillion to one.

What was the reason—excuse, really—that the Carter administration used to stop reprocessing? It was *the threat of terrorism*. Let's consider briefly the problems from the standpoint of terrorists who are planning a heist of plutonium, with which they intend to make a bomb.

There Has Just *Got* to Be a Better Way

Anyone who has the slightest familiarity with nuclear power knows that it is impossible to steal fuel from an operating reactor. Even assuming a terrorist knew how to shut it down, there is still the problem of very high level radiation within the reactor core that would be fatal in a matter of minutes for anyone who attempted to break in. (Our brave terrorist—pardon the oxymoron—would find this a very unpleasant way to enter paradise.)

The same goes for hijacking the spent-fuel truck or train on the way to the reprocessing plant. After storage for at least five years at the power plant site, the "spent" fuel is still highly radioactive and thermally quite hot. Hijacking 44,000-pound fuel containers— designed to smash into a concrete wall at 60 mph or fall onto a spike from thirty feet without rupturing—is a bit difficult to do surreptitiously.

This leaves us with raiding the reprocessing plant (bad idea) or stealing the fuel from shipments to the power plant (best bet). Assuming that the militants can make off with a huge truck, monitored as all valuable shipments are with global positioning electronics and probably guarded, and that no one notices this cargo with the huge radioactive symbols all over it, the hijackers must plan ahead to make sure their plutonium reclamation plant is near by. Typically the price tag on such a facility is in the hundreds of millions, or billions of dollars—and, of course, they've got to hide this construction from the prying eyes of swarms of government inspectors looking for something to inspect…or, even more difficult to avoid, the office-supply salesmen in the four surrounding counties.

Assuming the truck is hijacked and taken to the secret $100 million facility, the problems are just starting for our ill-intentioned thieves. Now they must cut up the fuel assemblies and dissolve them in nitric acid. After that, the chemical processes to separate

---

[4] A combination of uranium and plutonium oxides.

the plutonium from the uranium are devilishly tricky—in part because an almost-certainly fatal *criticality accident* can occur quite easily when the plutonium is in a liquid form. But let's assume that our "clever" terrorists are successful in refining out the plutonium and have shaped it for a bomb. Two big problems:

The first is obtaining the explosive charges necessary to "implode" a sphere of plutonium in on itself—essentially taking a hollow globe and compressing it down to a golf or tennis-ball-sized solid...well, almost solid. Regular explosive won't work, as the charge must have different characteristics as it "burns" to maintain the shape of the shock wave that is doing the compressing. Then there is the matter of the initiator, or trigger—the device that produces a stream of neutrons to start the reaction inside a one-tenth microsecond envelope when they are needed. This was considered by the Manhattan Project team (approximately 130,000 personnel, including arguably the best physicists and engineers in the world) as one of the most difficult items to design. Polonium 210 and beryllium must be mixed thoroughly—but this must occur within the aforementioned 0.0000001-second time frame. But let's suppose they are able to do all this. Sorry, still no cigar.

For you see, problem two, the plutonium they liberated from the Imperialist Yankee Running Dogs is not suitable for making a decent bomb. Since BWR and PWR reactors "burn" fuel slowly, Pu239 is created not only from the U238, but also from the Pu240 isotope. While not a fissionable isotope (which wouldn't make much difference in small concentrations), it is a *spontaneous neutron emitter*, which bodes ill for aspiring bomb makers. Even a very small amount of Pu240 is sufficient to throw off the timing of the necessary bomb reaction by starting it before the implosion is complete—causing the bomb to fizzle. Oh, you'll get an explosion of sorts—perhaps sufficient to flatten a city block or two—but not as awful as what you could do with ammonium nitrate and a little fuel oil, à la Oklahoma City. (The 1947 Texas City blast—where

512 were killed—was also a fertilizer explosion, which didn't require any plutonium at all.)

Terrorists are, in my mind, among the most despicable of humankind. But this isn't to say they are stupid. If they want to kill people and spread fear, there are a lot of easier ways to do this, and they know it. Poisoning the water supply, blasting a hole in a dam, setting oil storage facilities afire when the wind is blowing toward a heavily populated area—the list goes on and on. But building a dud bomb from hijacked plutonium isn't one of them.

Five-Page Penalty for Delay of Book

Sorry to have spent so long on the subject of terrorism. It is far afield from hormesis and the positive applications of nuclear energy, but it is a false argument so often used by anti-nuclear people, and it is never refuted—or even questioned—in the media. We might note that our overseas neighbors know this "threat of terrorism" malarkey is total rot—but what do they care what *we* think? If it goes on long enough, they will be able to sell high-energy content products to us…while we lap up good old safe solar energy in our cotton fields. Suffice it to say that the "terrorists with the plutonium" excuse for stopping a major reprocessing facility is as thin as a dime—and worth far less.

Chapter 24
Yes, You Can Be Too Careful

Hundreds of billions of dollars are to be spent
'remediating' U.S. sites even though
there is no scientific basis for claiming
any health or other benefit.
—Theodore Rockwell

In 1988, AN EARTHQUAKE registering 7.9 on the Richter scale devastated Soviet Armenia, leaving more than 25,000 people dead. Four years earlier, in far more densely populated Mexico City, an 8.1 earthquake (with a 7.8 aftershock thirty-six hours later) killed 9,000 people.

Seven years after the Armenian quake, they were still trying to get electrical power to the cities for more than two hours per day; Mexican Power and Light restored power to its 3,200,000 customers in seventy-two hours.

While Mexico isn't exactly the most advanced country in our hemisphere, compared with the communist paradise of Armenia it is Beulahland. Its buildings were built to stronger, more earthquake-resistant standards; when people were trapped in collapsed buildings, there were tools to get them out, and power to run the tools. There were hospitals for the wounded, and sanitary conditions prevailed for the survivors. In short, Mexico *had a superior infrastructure and was richer* than Armenia. Its wealth saved the lives of thousands of people who would have otherwise died.

There have been many attempts to determine a reasonable estimate for the value of a human life in the United States. One of these I can remember set the figure at $20 million, contending that for every $20 million taken out of the economy, the lowered standard of living for all would cause the premature death of one person.[1] While I can't vouch for this particular figure, the Armenian-Mexican situation shows clearly that there is a relationship of this nature. And it may be logically inferred from this that government, by wasting or compelling others to waste money, has a detrimental effect on the well-being of its citizens.[2]

Theodore Rockwell, in an article "What's wrong with being cautious?"[3] suggests five different kinds of harm that originate in the Linear No-Threshold hypothesis:

- Billions of dollars wasted
- Ridiculous regulations imposed that degrade the credibility of science and government
- Destructive fear generated
- Detrimental health effects created
- Environmental degradation accelerated. (This final item refers to the incredible amount of ash and sludge—equal to about 100 truckloads per *day*—produced by a coal-fired 1,000 megawatt power plant, compared with less than a Volkswagen full per *year* of actual high-level wastes from an equal-sized nuclear plant.)

Rockwell gives an example of a forklift driver who moved a small spent fuel cask from the fuel-storage pool to another location. As the cask had not been completely drained prior to being moved, some water was dribbled onto the blacktop along the way. But since

---

[1] This sounds a lot like *collective dose* to me; except that we can—on occasions like Armenia—count the dead.

[2] In 1980, Congress commissioned the National Acid Precipitation Assessment Program, which was expected to show that the utilities were responsible for acid rain. It found, to the amazement of the scientists involved, that this was not true. But Congress, which had paid $500 million for the study, ignored it and mandated scores of billions of dollars in unnecessary "scrubbers" to remove an insignificant fraction of power-plant emissions. At $20 million per life, politicians killed hundreds with this single vote.

[3] From *Nuclear News*, June 1997. A large part of this chapter is blatantly taken from this excellent article.

storage pool water is defined as a *hazardous contaminant*—by the regulators, not plant employees who had earlier used the pool for unauthorized midnight swims—it was deemed necessary to dig up the entire path of the forklift, some two feet wide by one-half mile long. It doesn't stop here.

Because the paving contractor used thorium-rich slag from a local phosphate plant as aggregate in the new pavement, it was *more* radioactive than the material that had been dug up—which was marked with the ominous radiation symbol and hauled away for expensive, long-term burial. Fortunately, it was only taxpayers' money.

Bernard Cohen reports, in his book *The Nuclear Energy Option*,[4] that $100,000 in medical treatments or highway safety improvements would save a life. Government, meanwhile, spends—or requires the spending of—$2.5 billion (yes, that's *billion*) to save a life from radiation exposure at the cost of 25,000 less "obvious" lives. And it now appears that the life supposedly saved from low-level radiation wasn't saved at all, as it is surfacing that the decrease in hormetic range radiation is actually costing lives.

Another appalling case reported by Rod Adams, editor of *Atomic Energy Insights,* involved a project used to blast out "contaminated soil" near the nuclear reactor at McMurdo Sound in Antarctica. Battling potentially lethal weather conditions, the task was completed at considerable risk to the workers and immense cost to taxpayers. So what was done with the offending material that may have caused a needed hormetic effect in the radiation-poor polar region? It was shipped (at another obscene cost to the taxpayers) to the United States, where it was used for parking lot fill in Port Hueneme, California.

Rather than trying to paraphrase the flowing and informative prose of Dr. Rockwell, here is a final example of government's mindless adherence to the Linear No-Threshold hypothesis—in his words:

---

[4] Plenum Press, New York, 1990.

The question of whether tiny amounts of radiation must be avoided, even at great cost, is neither abstract nor trivial. Hundreds of billions of dollars are to be spent "remediating" U.S. sites even though there is no scientific basis for claiming any health or other benefit. Worldwide, this cost has been estimated at more than a trillion dollars.[5] This is in addition to the unquantifiable cost of lives lost by fear of mammograms, radioactive smoke detectors, irradiated food, or other beneficial uses of radiation. Most, if not all, of this cost would be saved if we did not try to reduce radiation levels below the natural radiation background, which is several hundred times lower than the lowest levels at which any health effects have been found.

Rockwell continues,

But one person's wasted tax money is another's lucrative contract. Here's one example to remember. At some 46 sites in 14 states, there are some 82 million cubic feet of uranium tailings left over from the wartime weapons program. This material is what is left when you take as much uranium out of the natural ore as you can. *It is now less radioactive than the original ore, and 20 times less radioactive than what the law calls "low-level waste." There is a lot of natural rock that is more radioactive.* [Emphasis added.]

The Dawn Mining Company was recently licensed to haul 35 million cubic feet of this material from the East Coast to a huge pit at its closed uranium mine near Ford, Washington. The material will travel to Spokane by train, then be transferred to trucks for the trip to the final destination. The company says this will require about 40 very large trucks, with six to nine axles and weighing 93,000 pounds each when loaded. These trucks will travel over the back roads each day for 260 days a year for five to seven years.

---

[5] A more recent estimate, based on actual remediation projects, is $3 trillion worldwide, and $1 trillion for the United States alone. Using the figure of $20 million per life sacrificed, a trillion dollars is equal to 50,000 lives at the shrine of the Linear No-Threshold hypothesis.

Of course this doesn't include the expense of maintaining the roads under this unplanned-for load and the cost of the statistically certain accidents that will result from 93,000 pound trucks traveling some 5 million miles. But if you weren't lucky enough to get this contract, don't fret. There are another 47 million cubic feet of this material at other locations across the country. While you won't be producing any beneficial health effects, nobody really cares…and it's just taxpayers' money.

Even our state officials charged with insuring the public health are rebelling against the EPA and other heavy-handed federal government intrusions that have the force of law. For example, the EPA limit on radium-226 in drinking water is 5 pCi/l (0.18 Bq/l). The average adult will consume about one liter of water per day. Is there any evidence that 6 pCi/l will harm you? Not a whit. Yet to remove the radium is an expensive proposition borne by the local citizenry for an arbitrary, bureaucratic caprice.[6]

What evidence *is* there concerning the harm of ingested radium—in addition to the fact that people have been drinking the water for hundreds of years without ill effect?

There is good evidence of a death from radium about sixty years ago. But it wasn't from drinking water with 6 pCi/l.

In 1928, an eccentric millionaire, Eben Byers, was so enthusiastic about the invigorating qualities of a radium-based patent medicine that he partook of three to four vials per day of Radithor. Each vial contained 3,500,000 pCi of radium—a 1,918-*year* supply according to the EPA's limitations. He eventually died of his addiction after ingesting an estimated 10 billion pCi—a 5,480,000-year dose consumed in three years.

Eben isn't the whole story, however. There were 400,000 to 500,000 vials of Radithor sold with no indication that it caused any

---

[6] A South Carolina rural water district manager recently told me that one of their wells tested at 5.6 pCi/l, requiring special treatment at a cost of $30,000 per year to the customer base for that single well.

problems whatsoever. With what other "poison" can you consume 700,000 times the government-dictated maximum dose and still walk away...not once, but on a regular basis? Could the poison be in the dose?

While support for the LNT and collective dose is rapidly waning in light of the evidence brought forth by Luckey, Cohen, and a growing flood of researchers, there are still those who will (or perhaps feel they *must*) defend these hypotheses. Do they do so with evidence, such as dose-response curves? Not once have I seen low-level evidence showing an increased risk—unless it was an extrapolation from high-level data. The response is invariably the same: It is better to err on the side of safety than to take any chances on the possibility of an increased cancer risk.

If you're building a bridge, it doesn't cost much to increase its safety factor; a little more steel and concrete will do the trick. But the same doesn't go when building an airplane, as too great an emphasis on structural safety factors would keep the airplane from ever getting airborne. Regulators and bureaucrats—who are willing to see nuclear technology and hormesis research stay on the ground rather than expend the effort required to give a proper analysis to the overwhelming amount of data pointing to the threshold/hormesis models—are doing a great disservice to those whom they claim to be safeguarding. Whenever any of them starts feeling complacent about their rules and how they might be helping to save some theoretical life somewhere, I wish they would think a few seconds about a number—the number 100,000.

That's the lower estimate of unborn children who were aborted out of a totally unreasonable fear of their being "nuclear monsters." I wonder if those (almost) mothers sacrificed any Mozarts or Madame Curies or Salks on the altar of the LNT?

Chapter 25
Overcoming Vested Interests

*Bureaucracy defends the status quo long past
the time when the quo has lost its status.*
—Dr. Laurence J. Peter

IN LIGHT OF THE available evidence showing either the hormesis model or a threshold below which no harm occurs, it is difficult to understand why anyone would cling to the LNT hypothesis. This question was addressed at the 1999 Tucson Waste Management Conference in Stanley Logan's paper, "Radiation Exposure: Overcoming Vested Interests That Block Good Science."[1] After outlining the evidence for a re-evaluation of the entire radiation protection mechanism, Dr. Logan[2] defined the following groups that oppose or ignore evidence pointing away from the LNT and collective dose theories.

The Anti-Nuclear Camp

The anti-nuclear zealots will go to any lengths to preserve the myth that "no level of radiation exposure is safe." Their tactic is often to use ridiculous anecdotes ("fish so radioactive they glowed in the dark") to incite fear in the technically ignorant.

More than twenty years ago, I was present when the minions of Dr. Benjamin Spock were "debating" representatives of Arkansas Power and Light.[3] It was a rout. Spock's activists had no idea of the

---

[1] While I have borrowed heavily from Dr. Logan, I have embellished his material with my comments. In essence, the facts are his, the opinions are mine.

[2] Stanley E. Logan is founder of the Sante Fe consulting engineering firm that bears his name. A former associate professor of nuclear engineering, Dr. Logan has 27 years experience in areas of hazardous waste management and probabilistic risk analysis.

[3] Arkansas Power and Light was then owner of Arkansas Nuclear One—a complex with two 1,000-megawatt nuclear power plants.

reactor contents or of any way to begin quantifying the potential dangers of the plant. But they knew how to frame the debate: It was all about greedy industrialists intentionally endangering children, the elderly, the handicapped, the fishermen on the river, even birds flying over. Indeed, no one was safe from attack by this ruthless, rapacious cartel of profit mongers. Each accusation by Spock's forces brought forth wild cheers and applause.

The utility representatives were reduced to looking at each other with mouths open and eyes rolling. They came prepared to talk about containment building integrity and cesium 137—but not about *their war* on the community. When anyone from the nuclear camp dared to open his mouth, it was to a chorus of boos and heckling.

When the bloodbath was over, the anti-nukes marched out of the meeting as a cheering horde; the physicists and engineers were still sitting in shock when I left. Attempts to use a logical technical argument with this anti-nuclear group reminded me of trying to teach a pig to sing: It frustrates you and annoys the pig.

The Radon and Remediation Industries

One of the fascinating features of the free market is an almost instant appearance of entrepreneurs to fill a perceived need. Whether it is someone to build a skyscraper, supply illegal drugs, produce a million automobiles or a pornographic Mother's Day card—where there's a market, someone will appear to satisfy it. When the Environmental Protection Agency (EPA) recommended that you "fix the home if the radon level is 4 picocuries per liter or higher," it didn't take long for the "fixers" to step forward. Not just the fixers either; someone had to measure the radon, someone else had to build the instrumentation, others had to process the canisters, and still others had to evaluate the whole process. Soon an entire industry was created—and there is certainly nothing wrong with that. It's what we often term "the American way."

Because of their common interest, some of the parties involved in radon detection and remediation (mostly small businesses) joined together in an organization—the American Association of Radon Scientists and Technologists, Inc. (AARST)—and there certainly isn't anything wrong with that, either. But let us look at a little problem caused by the inherent ability of human beings to rationalize when their personal interests are at stake. Would the four or five hundred members of the AARST applaud an investigation to determine whether residential radon is actually a danger—or that it might possibly be a bio-positive agent for human health? Some probably would, and might then turn their attention to ways to get *more* radon in the residences, but most—I suspect—would do all in their power to prevent any such investigation.

So here we have a case where a few thousand highly motivated protectors of the status quo might be able to thwart an investigation that could be highly beneficial to hundreds of millions of uninformed—indeed, unaware—citizens. This is the basic reason that science, when politicized, is no longer science at all—but merely an extension of actions that enrich one group at the expense of another.

Regulatory Agencies

There are a number of national and international regulatory agencies (not to mention state, county, and municipal affiliates) whose entire reason for existence is to measure, verify measurement, and regulate levels of ionizing radiation. If the radiation hazard is defined as a linear relationship between radiation dose and effect (the LNT theory), then the job is relatively straightforward. But abandonment of the LNT would mean tossing most reference books, revising all the charts, and taking down the ubiquitous posters with such catchy phases as "Every Gamma Ray Can Be a Killer" or "Do You Really Need an X-ray?"

Given an understanding of low-level effects, many government agencies involved in such "non-protection" might mercifully go down the tubes; but for the technicians who have been working in the radiation environment, there may well be a silver lining. It is they who understand the mechanics of radiation—so who better to become operators or partners in the "hormesis clinics" that would undoubtedly spring up once the beneficial effects of low-level radiation were known? ("Good morning, Mrs. Jones, would you be interested in our special on two rads of deep therapy X-rays today for $225? It comes with a bonus of an hour in the 200 pCi per liter arthritis-relief chamber.")

As mentioned earlier, when one is looking forward to retirement, retraining is not a gratifying option—but what is the choice here? It is job security for a few people (who are, incidentally, quite employable) versus the continued enslavement of us all to a lie posing as science: the LNT hypothesis. At issue are the lives of all those who will die by following the LNT theory. Eventually, the truth will prevail—and we should continue to ask, "Why not now, rather than later?"

Risk Analysts and Others in the Nuclear Field

The LNT theory and the concept of collective dose make it relatively straightforward for assessors to determine the risk of exposure to radiation. There is only one problem with this currently accepted method: for the levels of radiation with which they are normally concerned, the results are meaningless—or worse.

As we have seen again and again, a wealth of hormesis data indicates not only that the current assessments of low-level dose-response are wrong in magnitude—but also in *sign,* with increasing amounts of radiation causing a decrease in harmful response. Would acknowledgement of this fact cause an upheaval in the risk business or what? Instead of "radiation = bad," they'd have to contend with "low radiation = good, but high radiation = bad"—and, moreover, have to determine when the "low and good" became "high and bad."

Risk analysts have about the same problems noted above for regulators—and for a very good reason: regulations are made from risk assessments.

Other Factors?

While Logan lists the groups that he believes have an aversion to even considering the possibility of a new regulatory structure, I've got a few more groups and other factors that I'll list by motivation:

1. Inertia. When most of us make a mistake, we own up to it and try not to make that mistake again. But it is different for scientists whose opinions are their stock in trade. Once some people take a position and harden it (and scientists are included in "some people"), they will take a conviction to the grave rather than admit they have been wrong.

2. Money. There are on-going and proposed projects that are based almost entirely on the LNT theory and collective dose. An example is Yucca Mountain—where scores to hundreds of scientists are engaged in the nuclear version of determining the number of angels who can dance on the head of a pin. Many of these scientists are among the smartest, kindest, nicest people on earth. Yet they intend to milk this cash cow for all its worth. (I understand this quite well, as I was in the NASA cow-milking business as a young engineer in the early 1960s.)

Suppose you are an associate professor at Armadillo State University, and your physics department head is on course for a $20 million federal contract to determine the safety of using residential smoke detectors. Are you going to blow the whistle and tell the grant committee that there are already data showing those devices are already completely safe? Oh *sure* you are—and you'll no doubt enjoy the sight of your effigy twisting in the wind from the lamppost in front of the physics building.

You remember the game: paper covers rock, rock breaks scissors, scissors cut paper. In federally sponsored research, politics covers truth.

3. The Good Old Boy Network. The National Fire Prevention Association is a non-government committee that seeks to minimize fire hazards in the United States. A subcommittee of this organization supervises the National Electric Code—or, in the parlance of all electricians, *the Code.* This subcommittee, which maintains and modifies *the Code* is made up of scientists, engineers, and master electricians. It also includes electrical contractors, users, manufacturers, and fire department officials—virtually everyone who is involved in the electrical industry. They are selected by an elaborate system that—while its primary function is to ensure safety and minimize fire risk—also recognizes advances in scientific knowledge, improvements in insulation and other materials, and new techniques that deliver electrical power safely and more efficiently. Without the NFPA and NEC, government-controlled agencies might still be requiring cloth insulation, fuse boxes, and pull chains on all lights. The NEC allows innovators to get their say, too.

Unfortunately, in the nuclear-safety business, there are no such safeguards to keep a relatively small number of LNT believers—connected through interlocking protection organizations, universities, and government agencies—from setting the regulation criteria. Independent observers and commercial interests not in the club need not apply.

Theodore Rockwell gives specifics of "good old boy networking" in regard to the selection process for the Biological Effects of Ionizing Radiation Committee:

> Most members have connections with the NRC, NCI, and/or EPA. Six members have served with NCRP, five with RERF, four with ICRP, one with BEIR, and one with NRPB. This is the same clique that has produced all the previous reports defending the status quo.

This is not a group capable of producing the "independent, impartial review" called for by the American Nuclear Society.[4]

Individual Action

So you're interested in seeing an honest re-evaluation of the effects of low-level radiation. What to do? Of course, buying and distributing huge quantities of this book would be my first choice, but there are others. If you are a member of a professional organization such as the Health Physics Society, write the president with copies to the other officers giving your opinion. There are organizations where the officers are very much behind the movement to bury the LNT theory but keep a low profile because of the "you've got to be kidding" response they tend to get on the subject. As knowledge of the subject becomes more widespread, more leaders are likely to become involved in the debate.

It may seem trite, but in this matter, writing your congressman and senators may have an effect. (Letters that *don't* start out "Why hasn't the government sent me my [fill in the benefit]…" get more attention because of their rarity.) As the debate heats up over the next months or years, an informative letter to your representative might even be appreciated.

Finally, this subject makes for a great letter to the editor. It is up to those of us who "know" to spread the word. With so much at stake, it is a timely and noble cause.

I leave you with my favorite quotation from one of the great physicists of the twentieth century, the late Nobel laureate Richard Feynman. He said it in 1965, long before the present controversy over the effects of low-level radiation, but certainly his words apply to today's battle with the false propositions of the LNT and collective dose:

---

[4] Quoted from personal correspondence from Theodore Rockwell to the author.

We look for a new law by the following process: first we guess at it. Then we compute the consequences of the guess to see what would be implied if this law we guessed is right. Then we compare the result of the computation with observation, to see if it works. If it disagrees with experiment, the law is wrong. In that simple statement is the key to science. It does not make any difference how beautiful your guess is. It does not make any difference how smart you are, who made the guess, or what his name is—if it disagrees with experiment, it is wrong. That is all there is to that.

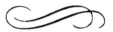

Epilogue

W<small>RITING A BOOK</small> seems to be much like building a house, where the final trimming and painting seems to take as much time as the rest of the project. I started this manuscript in 1998, and the first draft was complete in 2000. But then, because of personal circumstances, I was forced to put the book aside for several years. There was not a day during that period that I didn't kick myself for not getting this information out.

I mention this since you, dear reader, may have noted a dearth of studies and references after the year 2000. It is not because they're not there, but because if I had started over to include them, I never would have finished.

There are, however, several highlights during this time that I feel compelled to mention:

Microbiology

In chapter 10 (A Day or So in the Life of a Cell), it was noted that individual cells exposed to radiation *in vitro*, behaved as the LNT would predict: the more radiation, the less healthy the cell. And conversely when the cell was part of a system of cells (*in vivo*), the group of cells appeared to respond to radiation stimulation as a group—as if they were talking among themselves about the stimulus.

While I still have trouble believing it, there are now devices called "micro beams" that can shoot a single alpha particle into a particular cell. Along with this, there are methods to determine the chemical response to the target cell, as well as the cells in its vicinity. These experiments have clearly determined that cells do communicate—which we would suspect, as part of a complex organism requiring numbers of different types of specializations for survival. This confirms the existence of a mechanism known as the bystander effect, whereby a limited number of cells receiving a low dose can communicate a message to a large number of sibling cells.

International Recognition

In May 2005, the French Academy of Sciences and the National Academy of Medicine issued a *unanimous* report[1] that cut the legs from under both the LNT theory and collective dose. Regarding the former:

> In conclusion, this report doubts the validity of using LNT in the evaluation of the carcinogenic risk of low doses (< 100 mSv) and even more for very low doses (< 10 mSv). LNT can be a pragmatic tool for assessing the carcinogenic effect of doses higher than a dozen mSv within the framework of radioprotection. However the use of LNT in the low dose or dose rate range is not consistent with the current radiobiological knowledge.

In regard to collective dose:

> Decision-makers confronted with problems of radioactive waste or risk of contamination should re-examine the methodology used for the evaluation of risks associated with these very low dose exposures delivered at a very low dose rate. This analysis of biological data confirms the inappropriateness of the collective dose concept to evaluate population irradiation risks.

In the United States, June 2005 marked formal establishment of a technical society for the study of hormesis, both from radiation and chemical hormetins. The International Hormesis Society, a spin-off of the less specifically directed Biologically Effects of Low Level Exposures (BELLE) organization, is domiciled at the Univer-

---

[1] An English translation of the executive summary of this important report is given in its entirety in the appendix.

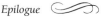

sity of Massachusetts, Amherst. You might want to visit its website at www.HormesisSociety.org. In 2006, it will take over and host the Fifth International Conference on Hormesis: Implications for Toxicology, Medicine, and Risk Assessment.

Cutting the Utility Power Cord

In the text of the book, I opined, "As far as I know, a low-power, inherently safe reactor has not been designed for community or home use" because of the risk to investors for such a project. That is no longer true. Toshiba calls its design the "4S reactor" for "super-safe, small and simple." It would be installed underground, and in case of cooling-system failure, heat would be dissipated through the Earth. There are no complicated control rods to move through the core to control the flow of neutrons that sustain the chain reaction. If the reflective panels are removed, the density of neutrons becomes too low to sustain the chain reaction.

Toshiba has offered to provide a compete nuclear power plant if the residents of the ice-bound 7,000-person town of Galena, Alaska, will but pay the operating costs—far less than the cost of barging diesel fuel in for the town generator. Will the anti-nuclear, primitivist-environmentalists be joyful because the townspeople won't be spilling diesel fuel during its arduous journey and will pay only a fraction of what they would pay for petroleum power? And because they won't be creating any of that pesky carbon dioxide that the environmentalists claim is warming the earth? Will they be grateful for the lack of long electrical transmission lines that somehow are sterilizing the caribou and ruining the vista for the six people that visit each year?

Certainly not. If nuclear power is *shown* to be as safe as it really is, then the anti-industrializers lose the only weapon they have to prevent a dynamically progressing civilization: their lies about an environmental apocalypse. Let us work to bring out the truth and have nuclear power in this remote village by 2010.

The Environmental Test Lab II

The unfortunate Japanese cities of Hiroshima and Nagasaki provide us with a test lab without peer. Thousands of citizens of all ages were exposed to different amounts of radiation in a very short period of time. From their locations at the time of the blast, their exposures could be determined with relative accuracy. Moreover, they were expected to carry and update their health records. As has been shown, the exposed survivors had unexpectedly longer and healthier lifetimes than did their unexposed cohorts.

But there is now a laboratory for low-level radiation absorbed over a period of twenty years. From 1982 to 1984, about 180 apartment buildings housing 10,000 Taiwanese tenants were built with cobalt-60-contaminated steel (half-life of 5.3 years). Since, as we all know, radiation causes cancer, these unfortunates must be dying like flies.

Well, not exactly. The assessed cancer rate of occupants of the apartments is 3.5 deaths per 100,000 person-years. The average death rate of the general population over the same twenty-year period is 116 persons per 100,000 person-years—resulting in a 97% *reduction* of fatal cancer.

Have you heard about this story on *Headline News*? No? Well, maybe no one is interested in reducing his risk of cancer by ninety-seven percent. But just in case you are, you may want to take a look at a paper entitled, "Is Chronic Radiation an Effective Prophylaxis Against Cancer?"[2]

Chernobyl Revisited

Let us return to mankind's worst nuclear disaster, Chernobyl. We have been told that the embryos and children in the downwind plume of extremely radioactive materials would be mutated. A

---

[2] Chen, W.L., Luan, Y.C., et al., "Is Chronic Radiation an Effective Prophylaxis Against Cancer?" *Journal of American Physicians and Surgeons,* Vol. 9, No. 1, Spring 2004. Taiwanese officials have resisted providing information needed for a first rate epidemiological report, apparently embarrassed that their LNT predictions didn't pan out.

recent report, which I was pleased to hear radio commentator Paul Harvey bring to the attention of his vast listening audience, found that the children of Chernobyl—eighteen years after the accident— were indeed showing effects, but *not* the type that were expected:

> The Chernobyl nuclear disaster has spawned a generation of "mutant" super brainy children. Kids growing up in areas damaged by radiation from the plant have a higher IQ and faster reaction times, say Russian doctors. They are also growing faster and have stronger immune systems. Radiation from the Ukrainian Chernobyl plant swept the globe and affected more than seven million people.
>
> Professor Vladimir Mikhalev from Bryansk State University has tracked the health of youngsters growing up in areas hit by the fallout since the 1986 accident. He compared their mental agility and health to those in unaffected area and found they came out tops in tests.[3]

Obviously, this has nothing to do with mutations—only the predictable result of radiation hormesis.

The "Linear Mafia's" Last Hurrah?

On June 29, 2005, a politicized committee appointed by the National Academy Sciences issued a well-publicized report that is in total disagreement with the unanimous French Academy of Science and Academy of Medicine's May 2005 report. H. Josef Hebert, an Associated Press writer,[4] summarized its conclusions:

> The preponderance of scientific evidence shows that even very low doses of radiation pose a risk of cancer or other health problems

---

[3] As reported in the British newspaper *The Sun,* on May 26, 2005, as well as in the Russian newspaper *Pravda,* on May 24, 2005. The story was—not surprisingly—virtually ignored in the mainstream media.

[4] As printed in the *Arkansas Democrat-Gazette,* Little Rock, Ark., June 30, 2005, p. 2.

and there is no threshold below which exposure can be viewed as harmless, a panel of prominent scientists concluded Wednesday.

The finding by the National Academy of Sciences panel is viewed as critical because it is likely to significantly influence what radiation levels government agencies will allow at abandoned nuclear power plants, nuclear weapons production facilities and elsewhere.

The nuclear industry...as well as some independent scientists, have argued that there is a threshold of very low level radiation where exposure is not harmful, or possibly even beneficial. They said current risk modeling may exaggerate the health impact.

The panel, after five years of study, rejected that claim.

Needless to say, this report was met with outrage by the scientists who have incontrovertible evidence to the contrary— evidence that was simply ignored by a panel of the same Good Old Boys who held to the LNT hypothesis on earlier requests to examine the accumulating evidence. The reaction of Gerald Looney, M.D., a California physician, is typical:

The medical profession is fully in favor of progress, but change is out of the question! I am embarrassed and frustrated by the rigid and reactionary viewpoints of my colleagues. Today's report carries the conclusion of a NAS panel of people who are old enough to know better but continue to support and promulgate the patently false Linear No-Threshold (LNT) hypothesis of radiation risk....

Perhaps this myopic view could be tolerated a while longer, except that it has an increasingly harmful impact on future generations. The current public (and panel) phobia of even a single ionizing ray leads to an expectation of zero tolerance from current environmental and political leaders. Such fear and intolerance makes us easy prey and our cities potential and prolonged wastelands in the face of even a small dirty bomb producing a tiny and harmless, but definitely measurable, increased level of radioactivity over a wide

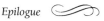

area, thereby allowing a terrorist to literally hoist us on our own petard.

The doctor also has a frightening personal story to tell. He and his partner Nancy were scheduled for the type of whole-body scans (WBS) that the NAS panel's report recommends be avoided. Nancy took the advice of scientific colleagues who suggested she beware of ionizing radiation inherent in CT scans. Unfortunately, an asymptomatic cancer was already under way, and the lack of early treatment proved fatal. Dr. Looney was to take the scan, resulting in a cancer's being found on his kidney. That cancer was surgically removed, apparently successfully.

Concerning the phobic position of the NAS, Dr. Looney writes:

> Public and professional policy, even when it comes from the National Academy of Sciences, seems clearly erroneous when a patient follows their official guidelines and advice but succumbs to curable pathology, while another patient ignores these same policies and thereby survives similar disease.

We began in the prologue with the sacrifice of my sister's fetus to an ignorance of low-level radiation effects, and we end with an avoidable death resulting from similar ignorance. Along the way, we saw, among many similar increases in life span and health, that a dose of 0.15 Gy would likely prevent 10,000 breast cancer deaths—with better than 99% certainty—if given to a million women.

How many more lives must be forfeited to a thoroughly discredited LNT before reason prevails?

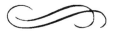

Appendix

 Académie des Sciences [Academy of Sciences]
Académie nationale de Médecine
[National Academy of Medicine]

Dose-effect relationships and estimation of the carcinogenic effects of low doses of ionizing radiation

March 6, 2005

André Aurengo[1] (Rapporteur), Dietrich Averbeck, André Bonnin,[1] Bernard Le Guen, Roland Masse,[2] Roger Monier,[3] Maurice Tubiana1[3] (Chairman), Alain-Jacques Valleron,[3] Florent de Vathaire

Executive Summary

The assessment of carcinogenic risks associated with doses of ionizing radiation from 0.2 Sv to 5 Sv is based on numerous epidemiological data.

However, the doses which are delivered during medical X-ray examinations are much lower (from 0.1 mSv to 20 mSv). Doses close to or slightly higher than these can be received by workers or by populations in regions of high natural background irradiation.

Epidemiological studies have been carried out to determine the possible carcinogenic risk of doses lower than 100 mSv and they have not been able to detect statistically significant risk even on large cohorts or populations.

Therefore these risks are at worst low since the highest limit of the confidence interval is relatively low. It is highly unlikely that putative carcinogenic risks could be estimated or even established for such doses through case-control studies or the follow-up of

---

[1] Membre de l'Académie nationale de médecine

[2] Membre correspondant de l'Académie nationale de médecine

[3] Membre de l'Académie des Sciences

cohorts. Even for several hundred thousands of subjects, the power of such epidemiological studies would not be sufficient to demonstrate the existence of a very small excess in cancer incidence or mortality adding to the natural cancer incidence which, in non-irradiated populations, is already very high and fluctuates according to lifestyle. Only comparisons between geographical regions with high and low natural irradiation and with similar living conditions could provide valuable information for this range of doses and dose rates. The results from the ongoing studies in Kerala (India) and China need to be carefully analyzed.

Because of these epidemiological limitations, the only method for estimating the possible risks of low doses (< 100 mSv) is by extrapolating from carcinogenic effects observed between 0.2 and 3 Sv. A linear no-threshold relationship (LNT) describes well the relation between the dose and the carcinogenic effect in this dose range where it could be tested. However the use of this relationship to assess by extrapolation the risk of low and very low doses deserves great caution. Recent radiobiological data undermine the validity of estimations based on LNT in the range of doses lower than a few dozen mSv which leads to the questioning of the hypotheses on which LNT is implicitly based: 1) the constancy of the probability of mutation (per unit dose) whatever the dose or dose rate, 2) the independence of the carcinogenic process which after the initiation of a cell evolves similarly whatever the number of lesions present in neighboring cells and the tissue.

Indeed 1) progress in radiobiology has shown that a cell is not passively affected by the accumulation of lesions induced by ionizing radiation. It reacts through at least three mechanisms: a) by fighting against reactive oxygen species (ROS) generated by ionizing radiation and by any oxidative stress, b) by eliminating injured cells (mutated or unstable), through two mechanisms i) apoptosis which can be initiated by doses as low as a few mSv thus eliminating cells whose genome has been damaged or misrepaired, ii) death at the time of mitosis cells whose lesions have not been repaired.

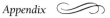

Recent works suggest that there is a threshold of damage under which low doses and dose rates do not activate intracellular signaling and repair systems, a situation leading to cell death c) by stimulating or activating DNA repair systems following slightly higher doses of about ten mSv.

Furthermore, intercellular communication systems inform a cell about the presence of an insult in neighboring cells. Modern transcriptional analysis of cellular genes using microarray technology reveals that many genes are activated following doses much lower than those for which mutagenesis is observed. These methods were a source of considerable progress by showing that according to the dose and the dose rate it was not the same genes which genes that were transcribed.

For doses of a few mSv (< 10 mSv), lesions are eliminated by the disappearance of the cells. For slightly higher doses damaging a large number of cells (therefore capable of causing tissue lesions), the repair systems are activated. They permit cell survival but may generate misrepairs and irreversible lesions. For low doses (< 100 mSv), the number of mutagenic misrepairs is small but its relative importance, per unit dose, increases with the dose and dose rate. The duration of repair varies with the complexity of the damage and their number. Several enzymatic systems are involved and a high local density of DNA damage may lower their efficacy. At low dose rates the probability of misrepair is smaller. The modulation of the cell defense mechanisms according to the dose, dose rate, the type and number of lesions, the physiological condition of the cell, and the number of affected cells explains the large variations in radiosensitivity (variations in cell mortality or probability of mutations per unit dose) according to the dose and the dose rate that have been observed. The variations in cell defense mechanisms are also demonstrated by several phenomena: initial cell hypersensitivity during irradiation, rapid variations in radiosensitivity after short and intense irradiation at a very high dose rate, adaptive responses which cause a decrease in radiosensitivity of the cells during hours or days following a first low dose irradiation, etc..

2) Moreover, it was thought that radiocarcinogenesis was initiated by a lesion of the genome affecting at random a few specific targets (proto-oncogenes, suppressor genes, etc.). This relatively simple model, which provided a theoretical framework for the use of LNT, has been replaced by a more complex process including genetic and epigenetic lesions, and in which the relation between the initiated cells and their microenvironment plays an essential role. This carcinogenic process is confronted by effective defense mechanisms in the cell, tissue, and the organism. With regard to tissue, the mechanisms which govern embryogenesis and direct tissue repair after an injury seem to play an important role in the control of cell proliferation. This process is particularly important when a transformed cell is surrounded by normal cells. These mechanisms could explain the lesser efficacy of heterogeneous irradiation, i.e., local irradiations through a grid as well as the absence of a carcinogenic effect in humans or experimental animals contaminated by small quantities of a-emitter radionuclides. The latter data suggest the existence of a threshold. This interaction between cells could also help to explain the difference in the probability of carcinogenesis according to the tissues and the dose, since the death of a large number of cells disorganizes the tissue and favors the escape from tissue controls of an initiated cell.

3) Immunosurveillance systems are able to eliminate clones of transformed cells, as is shown by tumor cell transplants. The effectiveness of immunosurveillance is also shown by the large increase in the incidence of several types of cancers among immunodepressed subjects (a link seems to exist between a defect in NHEJ DNA repair and immunodeficiency).

These phenomena suggest the lesser effectiveness of low doses, or even of a practical threshold which can be due to either a failure of a low level of damage to sufficiently activate DNA repair mechanisms or to an association between apoptosis + error-free repair +

immunosurveillance, to determine a threshold (between 5 and 50 mSv?). The stimulation of the cell defense mechanisms could also cause hormesis by fighting against endogenous mutagenic factors, in particular against reactive oxygen species. Indeed a meta-analysis of experimental data shows that in 40% of animal experiments there is a decrease in the incidence of spontaneous cancers after low doses.

This observation has been overlooked so far because the phenomenon was difficult to explain.

These data show that the use of a linear no-threshold relationship is not justified for assessing by extrapolation the risk of low doses from observations made for doses from 0.2 to 5 Sv since this extrapolation relies on the concept of a constant carcinologic carcinogenic effect per unit dose, which is inconsistent with experimental and radiobiological data. This conclusion is in contradiction with those of an article and a draft report [43,118], which justify the use of LNT by several arguments.

1. for doses lower than 10 mGy, there is no interaction between the different physical events initiated along the electron tracks through the DNA or the cell;
2. the nature and the repair of lesions thus caused are not influenced by the dose and the dose rate;
3. cancer is the direct and random consequence of a DNA lesion in a cell apt to divide;
4. LNT model correctly fits the dose-effect relationship for the induction of solid tumors in the Hiroshima and Nagasaki cohort;
5. the carcinogenic effect of doses of about 10 mGy is proven by results obtained in humans in studies on irradiation *in utero*.

With respect to the first argument, it should be noted that the physico-chemical events are identical but their biological consequence may greatly vary because the cellular defense reactions differ depending on dose and dose rate. The second argument is contradicted by recent radiobiological studies considered in the present report. The third argument does not take into account recent findings showing the complexity of the carcinogenic process and overlooks experimental data. Regarding the fourth argument, it can be noted that besides LNT, other types of dose-effect relationships are also compatible with data concerning solid tumors in atom bomb survivors, and can satisfactorily fit epidemiological data that are incompatible with the LNT concept, notably the incidence of leukemia in these same A-bomb survivors.

Furthermore, taking into account the latest available data, the dose-effect relationship for solid tumors in Hiroshima-Nagasaki survivors is not linear but curvilinear between 0 and 2 Sv. Moreover, even if the dose-effect relationship were demonstrated to be linear for solid tumors between, for example, 50 mSv and 3 Sv, the biological significance of this linearity would be open to question. Experimental and clinical data have shown that the dose effect relationship varies widely with the type of tumor and with the age of the individuals—some being linear or quadratic, with or without a threshold. The composite character of a LNT relationship between dose and all solid tumors confirms the invalidity of its use for low doses.

Finally, with regard to irradiation in utero, whatever the value of the Oxford study, some inconsistencies should lead us to be cautious before concluding to a causal relationship from data showing simply an association.

Moreover, it is questionable to extrapolate from the fetus to the child and adult, since the developmental state, cellular interactions, and immunological control systems are very different.

In conclusion, this report doubts the validity of using LNT in the evaluation of the carcinogenic risk of low doses (< 100 mSv) and even more for very low doses (< 10 mSv). LNT can be a pragmatic tool for assessing the carcinogenic effect of doses higher than a dozen mSv within the framework of radioprotection. However the use of LNT in the low dose or dose rate range is not consistent with the current radiobiological knowledge; LNT cannot

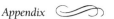

be used without challenge for assessing by extrapolation the risks of associated with very low doses (< 10 mSv), nor be used in benefit-risk assessments imposed on radiologists by the European directive 97–43. Biological mechanisms are different for doses lower than a few dozen mSv and for higher doses. The eventual risks in the dose range of radiological examinations (0.1 to 5 mSv, up to 20 mSv for some examinations) must be estimated taking into account radiobiological and experimental data. An empirical relationship which is valid for doses higher than 200 mSv may lead to an overestimation of risk associated with doses one hundredfold lower and this overestimation could discourage patients from undergoing useful examinations and introduce a bias in radioprotection measures against very low doses (< 10 mSv).

Decision makers confronted with problems of radioactive waste or risk of contamination, should re-examine the methodology used for the evaluation of risks associated with these very low dose exposures delivered at a very low dose rate. This analysis of biological data confirms the inappropriateness of the collective dose concept to evaluate population irradiation risks.

Acknowledgements

O<small>VER THE PAST</small> several years I have had occasion to attend seminars and conferences where I was able to meet personally with many of those I have quoted. Without exception, they have taken time for my often "dumb" questions and have encouraged me to help "create understanding" about hormesis and the invalidity of the LNT theory.

Don Luckey answered my questions for hours sitting in his den in Ft. Collins, Colorado. Bernie Cohen did the same in his office at the University of Pittsburgh. I met Myron Pollycove at a conference in Ottawa and had a long dinner with Ted Rockwell in Boston. I visited the Chalk River reactor facility at the invitation of Ron Mitchel. Ed Calabrese, the first director of the International Hormesis Society, welcomed me warmly to the Amherst symposium. All these men have doctorates in the hard sciences (Pollycove is an M.D.), and I must admit to being a bit intimidated when I first approached them. Their generous assistance has been appreciated more than they know.

I owe a special thanks to Massachusetts State Nuclear Engineer Jim Muckerheide. Jim—also the president of the non-profit organization Radiation, Science and Health—and his wife Linda have provided more information for this book than anyone, with the exception of Dr. Luckey. Their support has been invaluable.

Others who were willing to read and make technical comments on the draft manuscript include Michael Gough (then of the Cato Institute), health physicist Paul Beck, pathologist M.G. Simpson, physics professor emeritus Howard Hayden, and my old friend Ed Gran of the University of Arkansas at Little Rock physics department. Lastly, William R. Hendee, Ph.D., dean of the Graduate School of Biomedical Sciences at the Medical College of Wisconsin—not known for his support of the hormesis thesis—gave me valuable insights.

In the nontechnical area, I am indebted to the late Irene Beckmann, my sister Martha Johnson, and Jane Jacob for reading early drafts and making helpful suggestions and corrections.

So many others were helpful along the way, and I have been so lax about recording their names. To all of them, my earnest thanks.

And finally, many thanks to Laissez Faire Books for its support on this project.

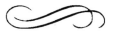

Index

F

Falling analogy 10

Finland 146

Fonda, Jane 51

France 8, 19, 105, 183, 224, 227, 231

 French Academy of Sciences 224, 227, 231

Free Enterprise Mine 157–159

Fusion 15, 191, 197–199

G

Gamma knife 149

Gamma radiation 17, 39–41, 43, 49, 54, 55, 58, 68, 75, 98, 100, 102, 105, 109, 113, 129, 149, 165, 197, 205, 217

Gamma rays
 (see Gamma radiation)

Gasteiner Heilstollen 88

General Adaptive Syndrome, The 26

Geothermal wells 18

Germany 146, 171

Gilbert, Ethel 126, 131

Global collective dose 11

Gofman, John 39, 41, 128

Goia 20–21, 196, 203

Graphite 20, 81, 82, 181

Gray 55, 58

Greece 7–8

Greens 2–3, 16, 93, 192

Gribbin, M.A. 124

Guarapari Beach (Brazil) 80, 144

Guinea pigs 61, 98

H

H-bomb 19, 76, 161, 193

Half-life 42–45, 50, 58, 76, 82, 85, 179, 195, 203, 226

Hanford Reservation (Washington) 12, 127, 195

Hattori, Sadao 159–160

Health handbook 113, 114

Health Physics 2

Health Physics and Radiological Health Handbook 11

Healthy worker effect (HWE) 122–123, 126, 130–131, 163, 166

Heavy water 183–184

Heiby, Walter 26

Hiroshima 20, 64, 113, 115, 116, 117, 160, 174, 226

Hoffman, Abby 7

Homeopathic Medicine (Hahnemann) 25

Homeostasis 72

Hormesis 3–4, 11–12, 14, 16, 23, 25–31, 53, 54, 62–65, 67, 71–72, 75, 86, 91–95, 97–98, 100, 102–106, 111, 115, 118, 121–123, 125–127, 130, 131, 140–142, 153–154, 156, 159, 163–164, 201, 203, 214, 215, 218, 224–225, 227

 Typical hormesis curve 28

Hormesis with Ionizing Radiation 3

Hormetins 26–28, 130, 224

Hormoligosis 26

Hosoi, Y. 102

HWE (see Healthy worker effect)

Hydrogen bomb (see H-bomb)